Table of Contents

Introduction

Everything that you have learned about fitness, health, losing weight, and getting proper nutrition is just plain wrong.

Organizations like health clubs and fitness centers, wellness facilities, hospitals, schools, supplement manufacturers, insurance and drug companies, government entities such as the USDA, CDC, NIH; professionals like personal trainers, nutritionists, and doctors, that are established or trained to help teach people what it is that they are supposed to do to have optimum health, fitness and nutrition, haven't the foggiest clue how to do it.

Exponential breakthroughs in science of how our body works at the cellular level have made defining the requirements needed for optimum health and wellness rather easy. If you get anything from this book, get this: there is a scientific revolution happening now that will impact our lives as much as the industrial revolution and the technical revolution that most of us have experienced in the last 25 years. Because of the technology revolution allowing scientists to see exactly what is happening in and around our cells has led to the scientific revolution that is happening now! If you can remember back to the little girl in the commercials in the early 1990's saying, "Are you ready? "Are you ready for the Information Super Highway?" You could feel the ground shaking and you knew exciting things were going to happen. Now I am asking you… "are you ready?" Get out your mind stretchers and hang on to your butts because what you perceive as possible today about your health and aging will be gone. It's all going to change.

Traditional methods for improving fitness, health, losing weight, and getting proper nutrition focus on how one looks, how one feels, or how big one's biceps are. Traditional medicine advocates surgery or drugs to cut out disease or cure disease by taking the right drug. The focus needs to be placed on the micro-mechanics and interconnections of what happens in the cells. By doing so, the understanding of how to develop a practical approach to deliver this new and exciting information and design a complete program that gets one results quickly, safely and continuously without taking enormous amounts of time is obviously understood by few.

1

"This book is not intended to criticize those that haven't got it right"

Just look around you: what we experience as normal health and aging isn't normal. 3 million people die in the United States alone from preventable diseases and ailments... EVERY YEAR! Who the next 3 million are going to be is obvious. You can see it in future generations. Our children eat poorly and are not active enough. If you understand what is possible, this outcome is a colossally pathetic attempt at living. It is almost like one has set this as a goal and works towards it everyday to achieving it. Imagine that everyone's life were a boat. We are all out there sailing around. We all have ups and downs, and one day we know that the boat is going to, over time, get too old to float, rot and will sink. I know that you wouldn't do this but, now imagine that there are a number of boat owners that have drills and you look over and notice that they are drilling holes in the bottom of their boats. "Big Ones," you say to yourself. "Huh, those boats are going to sink sooner than they have to." Then one guy stops and looks up at you and says (please read this with a gravelly voice), "We all gotta go sometime." He continues, "We all die of something, I would rather know what it is." You see the exact same thing going on when it comes to the diseases of aging. The only difference is that we don't - if we even notice - say anything. One takes the miracle of life and all its amazing systems, developed over millions of years, and totally neglects it. (Yes, use the voice), "I finally made it. I sat on my butt ate everything in sight. I was able to get heart disease, kidney disease, diabetes, my foot fell off from no circulation, I'm blind, have extremely high blood pressure, got cancer, stroked out at the age of 56, and spent the last 15 years of my life decrepit shuffling around behind a walker."

This book is written not to criticize those that haven't gotten it right. It is intended to offer an alternative for YOU to understand what is necessary for you to easily improve health, fitness, nutrition, and maintain an optimal weight without the worry of these dreaded diseases of aging creeping into your life. The great side effect of all of this is that you will look your best (slim, fit, and trim with a healthy glow). I am here to tell you that no matter who you are and what your circumstances are, you can change your state of being today and improve your chances by changing your lifestyle. The first step in changing your thoughts about who you are is getting the right information so that the confusion surrounding all this is cleared up for you. The second step is to begin to act upon that information. One needs

My intent is to describe this for you and bring a practical understanding of what is possible

to get up and do something intensely active for ½ hour per day. That's it! Do that and provide your cells what they need to work in symphony with each other so you are humming smoothly on all cylinders. The very areas of health that cause the biggest challenges to modern medicine are the areas that the human body seems very capable of improving itself when given the right signals, nutrients and Cellular Fitness.

For one that has never exercised before, this may be just walking for ½ an hour; for others who have been exercising for a while, it may mean upping the intensity so they continue to reap the benefits. My intent is to describe this for you and to bring to you a practical understanding of what is possible.

The book's inspiration comes from my father, Dr Robert A. Good.

Dad was born in Crosby, Minnesota on May 21, 1922, the second son of parents who worked as educators. The early death of his father from cancer was so devastating to him that he vowed to become a doctor and develop a cure for that dreadful disease in his lifetime.

With this added fuel he went on a quest for excellence. He attended the University of Minnesota, receiving his B. A. degree in 1944. While an undergraduate at the University of Minnesota, he developed a polio-like illness and entered medical school with his mother pushing him into classrooms in a wheelchair. Rebounding from this paralytic illness with characteristic vigor and boundless energy, he converted a pronounced limp into a trademark gait that always seemed to propel him forward. He developed a habit of working nearly 20 hours per day of every single day of his life and was the first to pursue combined PH.D and MD curriculum at the University of Minnesota. He did become that doctor when he was the first to earn his MD and PH. D. on the same day in 1947. His schedule was then used as the template for the combined curriculum PH.D./M.D. program still offered today at universities all over the world.

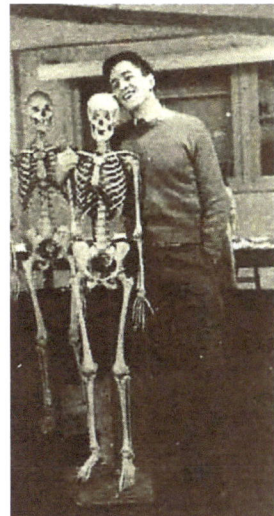

3

He is now regarded as the father of modern immunology

When Dr. Good began his research in immunology in 1944, we knew nothing of the cellular basis of immunity, little or nothing of the molecular basis of immunity, and did not have an inkling of the functions of the major organs of the lymphoid system such as the thymus gland, lymph nodes, and spleen. From 1944 to 1970, he studied and contributed to the understanding of how immunity works on the cellular level. From 1959 to 1979, he discovered the function of the thymus gland and thymic hormones. Dr. Good studied the two-component concept of immunology (1952-1969), immunodeficiency diseases (1975-1980), cellular engineering (1954-1980), and the effects of under-nutrition on aging (1985-2003). He authored more than 2,500 peer-reviewed scientific papers and abstracts and wrote more than 50 books, hundreds of other articles and received 75 honorary degrees and awards for outstanding contributions in medicine. He steadily contributed new knowledge and understanding of lymphoid cells, their functions, their cancers and malignancies, as well as to develop an entire school of scientists, each of whom has contributed and is continuing to contribute exciting discoveries to the understanding and analyses of the lymphoid systems and immunologic functions for the last 60 years.

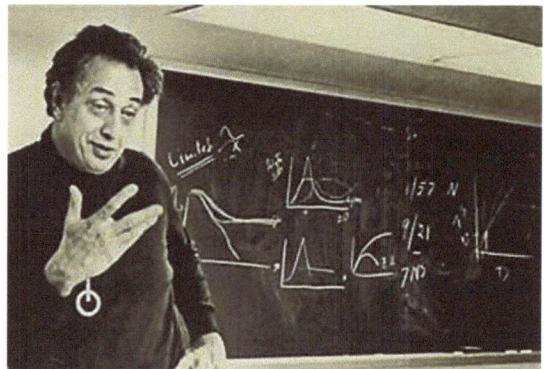

In 1968 Dr. Good used his concept of cellular engineering to perform the first successful human bone marrow transplant, on persons who were not identical twins. 8-month-old, David Camp was given bone marrow from his 9-year-old sister Doreen. This allowed David, a child with a rare deficiency in his immune system, who had no chance of living in Earth's sea of micro-organisms, to have bone marrow taken from one of his four siblings and transferred to him. This gave David a brand new immune system, and he was discharged from the hospital totally normal.

Dr. Good became one of the most influential immunologists of the 20th century. Robert Good's many contributions to understanding the cellular basis of immunity and immunodeficiency diseases made him the most

4

cited author in science from 1965 to 1978. He is now regarded as the father of modern immunology.

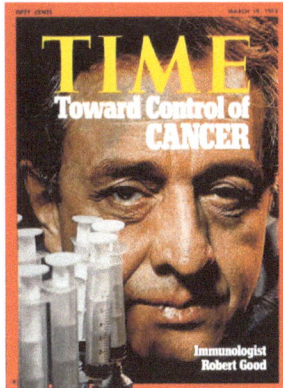

During this time, my two older brothers, two younger sisters, and I were growing up. I was particularly close with my dad. I had developed the habit of getting up early with him and over time we became quite good friends. He was my best friend. He used to get up at 4 AM every morning. I didn't get up as early as he did, but I usually was up before my siblings and that became a special time that I would bond with him. There were days when we would schedule a family outing together. He would get up at his usual time, get himself ready, take a bath, shave, and eat breakfast while we were sleeping. Then just as he was headed out the door he would click the light switch on and say, "come-on you guys, it's the crack of dawn." We would have to jump out of bed and be ready in minutes. He considered letting us sleep a little longer a favor to us and didn't realize that it was quite a shock to have to instantaneously go from a sound sleep to "come-on" mode. I did learn to get up quick. Now, I look back on those moments fondly. He always included us with his ideas about what his research was producing and was so enthusiastic about telling us of his discoveries and his thoughts about new things he was thinking. Times we went fishing and caught fish, he would dissect the fish before they were filleted and he would show us the fish's thymus gland, lymph nodes, appendix, spleen, and other organs and tell us about what he thought their functions, not known at the time, were.

Over time Dr. Good did, however, recognize that his crusade to cure cancer and the diseases associated with aging (heart disease, kidney disease, stroke, diabetes, and high blood pressure) was not the most practical approach. He recognized that it is a far more practical approach to prevent these diseases, and that people could extend their life span significantly by doing this. His research on aging across all experimental animal models consistently showed just by cutting their calories to a minimal level (under nutrition without malnutrition) that their lifespan quadrupled, and that extrapolating that to the human lifespan was probable.

There was an energy equation at work in the prevention of the diseases of aging

In 1984, Dr. Ralph Paffenbarger of Harvard established the significance of exercise for disease prevention, eliminating the diseases of aging, extending lifespan, and especially promoting the functioning of the immune system.

Dr. Good combined that proof with his understanding of under nutrition without malnutrition on how aging works and suggested that that there was an energy equation at work in the prevention of the diseases of aging, and that was all happening on the cellular level.

"As a pediatrician concerned primarily with the prevention of disease, I believe it is the manifest destiny of pediatrics to develop means to prevent all the diseases of adult life, including diseases of aging. A critical variable in preventing diseases is energy intake. Kidney disease, vascular disease, heart disease, and increased susceptibility to infection associated with aging all have been inhibited and prevented by the restriction of energy intake. The other side of the equation, energy utilization, also plays an important role in achieving a long life and good health. We discovered, in experimental models, that physical conditioning and regular strenuous exercise increases immunologic function. Exercise has been shown to have a favorable influence on the immunologic changes associated with aging, and cardiovascular disease, and it compliments our own research with calorie restricted diets where doubling tripling and quadrupling life span is done in all species. The influence on health of each component of this energy equation is impressive, but if both components can be taken together,

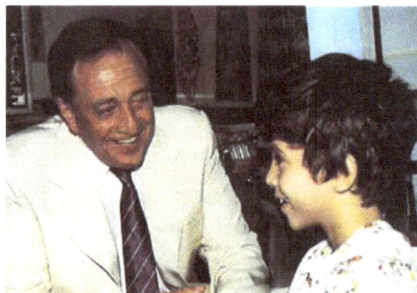

meaningful changes may be more easily applied than would be the case if only one side of the equation were concerned. Perhaps this approach will bring us closer to manifest destiny of pediatrics, the ability to prevent adult diseases and diseases of aging in humans."

If accidents were the only cause of death, man could live to be 600 years old

This just isn't a guess anymore. It is shown to be so and backed by scientific data. Furthermore it was the fitness of the cells "Cellular Fitness" that was really the key to understanding how this works and how practical it is.

When I was ready to graduate from high school, I had thoughts of what life would be like when dad passed. He had had his health problems when he was a young man, and I always was afraid that somehow it would affect his longevity. Having developed a close friendship, I asked him about it one day as were going to up Waverly Lake, Minnesota to go fishing with Hubert Humphrey. He told me that if he were to die tomorrow, that he would have no regrets. That he had lived a full life and that anything that happened onward would be a bonus. He lived another 30 years after that, and we only had one more conversation about that when he was in his 70s. He wanted to go over his assets and finances with me to inform me of the provisions that he had made for all of us. At that time I asked him with all the knowledge that he had accumulated and with his vision for the future, what would be the one thing that he could give me other than material possessions? He said without hesitation, "If accidents were the only cause of death, man could live to be 600 years old. That is not possible in my lifetime, but it is in yours." I then asked him: "at what point would science find everything there is to know?" He said, "Imagine, what we now know is like a pea in the corner of a large auditorium, and the rest of the room represents what we don't know."

Dad believed with great confidence that with the exciting revolutionary breakthrough advances happening now on a daily basis in medicine combined with lifestyle changes, that men and women could live productive lives free and clear of disease with vitality well beyond the benchmark of 100 years. That if heart and kidney disease, stroke, diabetes, cancer, and all diseases associated with aging could be prevented (leaving accidents as the only cause of death), then man could live to be 600 years old.

Chapter 1
Getting It Right

Everybody knows if you exercise, take vitamins and minerals "A" through Zinc, get all essential amino acids, eat and take antioxidants, eat fewer calories, lower cholesterol that it is all good for you. For the most part, however, people focus on the wrong things to get the results they want. They focus on building stronger muscles, losing weight, looking good, becoming "beach body beautiful," and taking drugs to lower blood pressure and cholesterol. Very few people are aware of the significant benefits of controlling body signals at the cellular level. The focus has to be put on "Cellular Fitness". If you shift your focus on to getting your cells fit, you can get the results you want, look your best, take control of your weight quickly, and stay healthy longer because that is where it all happens. It may be expressed in your physical appearance and in good numbers, but it ALL happens in the cells.

Most fitness and exercise programs use outdated methods and separate aspects into strength training, aerobics and flexibility programs. The problem with that approach is that the results are slow; the methods are dangerous and cause injuries. They take way too long for busy people to implement and are not intense enough to meet the necessary and definable requirements for your cells to be fit and deliver the benefit intended.

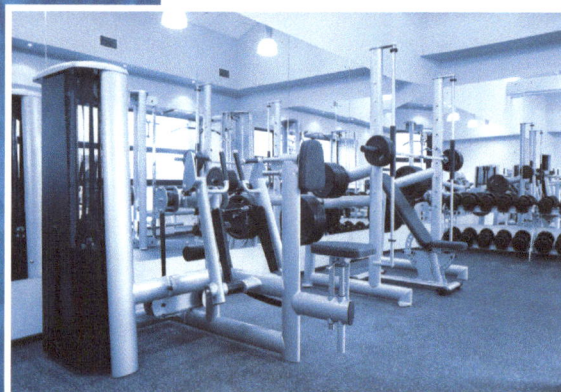

Health clubs and fitness centers bank on your paying for a membership. And they count on you not to use it. Most people who do use it think they are getting the benefit but either have a false belief, or are led to believe that they are getting the benefit when they are not. Either way, the only significant exercise that is happening is in the jaws and the lips. The only way to know if you are getting enough exercise is to know what that is and how to measure it. Walk in to any wellness or longevity center and ask them what one needs to do to live longer and be healthy. They will give you a blank stare or roll out the same old generic, "see your doctor, exercise, take vitamins, and eat right."

Most nutrition programs are designed around losing weight and dieting. Some focus on selling a particular product, an isolated nutrient, or eating low-calorie (loaded with salt) or fat-free food (loaded with sugar). Dr Soandso's has just come out with a new diet, just eat protein. Try Dr. Whatsandsuch's Diet, just eat carbohydrates. This approach has proven to be counter productive to one's health and basic biological cellular needs and never works long term.

The USDA compiles a collection of caliginous junk to appease commercial interests and then piles it into a "MyPyramid" of garbage, puts it on a "MyPlate," and serves it up to you as fact recommending you follow it.

Most health and health care programs designed recommend you do the above two things (exercise and diet) and then take drugs or have surgery to cure what isn't right and accept the fact, that you will dry up and blow away from 60 to 84... "We will take care of you." Doctors look to cure not to prevent. Most scoff at the suggestion that maybe if you get proper nutrition and exercise appropriately, most problems could be solved or prevented.

Schools administrators allow candy and soda machines in the schools for economic reasons and are shocked when many kids are overweight... Duh! Lunch room diets are the same old junk: full of salt, sugar, fat, and ice cream for dessert with no consideration to health guidelines.

Oh and what about the ever resounding noise that we are pounded 24/7 with the special powers supplier's products have that will make you healthy and trim easily. Eat Cheerios and lower your cholesterol; eat chocolate to get your flavonoids; Drink Diet Coke and become heart healthy; "One-A-Day Men's Vitamins maintain heart health and lowers your blood pressure"; Take vitamin A for great skin; "Hellman's Real Mayonnaise rich in omega 3"... get out the waders it's starting to get really deep! This is at best irresponsible, but unfortunately, it is where many people seem to be getting their information.

Let's also not forget the "hocus pocus" products like resveratrol, et. al. We live in an instant-coffee society where if what we want isn't simple and easy, we disconnect with it. We force ourselves to believe the easy way is the best way even though there is no evidence that it has any validity.

"Come on, Man!"

The hype one molecule can generate is truly amazing. That has been the fate of resveratrol: a substance found in red wine that some research suggests accounts for the cardiovascular and anti-aging benefits of red wine. Experiments in the early 2000s showed that resveratrol extended the life spans of yeast and other relatively simple organisms. Since then, media reports have extolled its virtues with headlines like "Fountain Of Youth In The Bottom Of A Wine Bottle" and "Want to slow down aging? Pop some red wine pills." Resveratrol for a longer life –works only if you're a yeast.

"Come on, Man!"

The alternative would be to design a program that is:

- Consistent and flexible with the new fantastic and dynamite scientific breakthrough information proved and backed by data

- Comprehensive to combine all aspects of exercise and fitness

- Combine all nutrients in their proper amounts and understand the dynamic interactive way that nutrients and systems complement each other on a cellular basis

- Make the program effective and efficient

- Educate on what the requirements are for optimum health so that all the confusion is eliminated

- Measure the results so that it is clear what the progress is

I have compiled a checklist so that you can make sure that you are getting everything that you require to live a long, healthy, vibrant life. If you follow this, you will be stronger, look your best, and be healthy longer.

See Checklist at the end of this book.

Chapter 2
Exercise Has To Be Intense Enough

I am well aware that only one person in a 1,000 will respond to this. Most people look for what is easy and quick. When confronted with evidence of what one has to do to get the results they want and it turns out to be too hard, they whine, complain, run and hide behind mommy's skirt like mamby pambies. If you are like most, maybe you should stop here and ask for a refund. If you happen to be the 1 in a 1,000 with the courage and guts to change the way you behave and are honest with where you are and really want to achieve your goals, I encourage you to continue. If you want to cut through the noise of misperceptions and downright lies that most have been holding near and dear to their hearts, then read on. If you do, you can have everything that you want. At the moment, only a fool would accept such a statement on absolute faith, without evidence whatsoever. But a wise man or woman, free of deadly self-limitation, would merely ask, "How?"

Go with me through these pages, step by step, and you will know!

When my brothers, sisters and I were growing up in Minnesota, we were all encouraged to pursue athletics. My sisters were younger and didn't seem to care for athletics much. My dad's three brothers were all very athletic and it rubbed off on us boys. My uncle Mick ran track, while attending medical school. He placed 4th in the US Olympic trials after studying all night for a final exam. Uncle Tom and Chuck were Champion Rowers. My dad was bigger, stronger, and more athletic than any of his siblings until he got his polio-like illness. He had learned to strive for excellence at a young age and instilled it in us. When his physicalness was taken from him, he turned his commitment for excellence toward his academics. He encouraged us to participate in sports because he got great pleasure seeing us succeed. Dad used to take us speed skating every night during the week, and we would compete every weekend during the winter months. We would pack up our skates and head down to the track

11

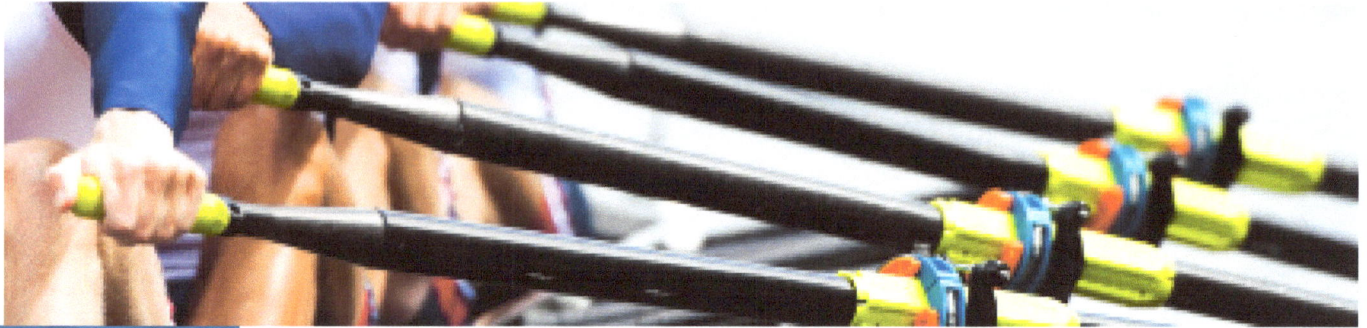

after school. His characteristic gait turned into an enthusiastic shuffle once he hit the ice, and he would stay outside with nothing more than a sweater for hours while we trained. His footwear was three pairs of socks and high-top Keds basketball sneakers that he called "tenny shoes." His attitude was upbeat and positive, and he always had a smile on his face. We would be bundled up, and, even though we were skating, we froze our butts off. I started skating at the age of three and initially cried through most of the workouts with cold feet, but by the age of 10, I had won the Minnesota State Indoor and Outdoor Speed Skating Championships. As I got older, my Uncle Chuck took me down to the Minneapolis Rowing Club and introduced me to the sport of rowing. After winning all the regional championships in the Midwest and graduating from the University of Minnesota in Wild Life Management, I was invited to row for the New York Athletic Club. Dr. Good was made President and Director of the Memorial Sloan Kettering Cancer Center in New York City and was also appointed as an advisor to President Nixon. So we moved to New York together. I then started my own fitness center in Westchester County, New York. It was a combination of free weights, Nautilus machines, and had a space for aerobic classes. I was able to support my athletic endeavors by running a successful business. I, concurrently, became head of fitness programming for the Sports Learning Corporation and developed "The Max Performance Programs."

I went on to win 21 National individual and team Championships in Rowing, represented the United States on 5 World teams, and placed 4th in the world. Our 8-oared crew team won the Elite Heavyweight Nationals Championships in 1980. Because Jimmy Carter boycotted the 1980 Moscow Olympics to, ironically, protest the Soviet's war in Afghanistan, we were not allowed to go to the Olympics.

Before 1984, exercise was only suspected to be good for you

Before 1984, exercise was only suspected to be good for you. There was a lot of enthusiasm about it. We knew it made you look better, was beneficial in helping you expend calories, losing weight, and made you

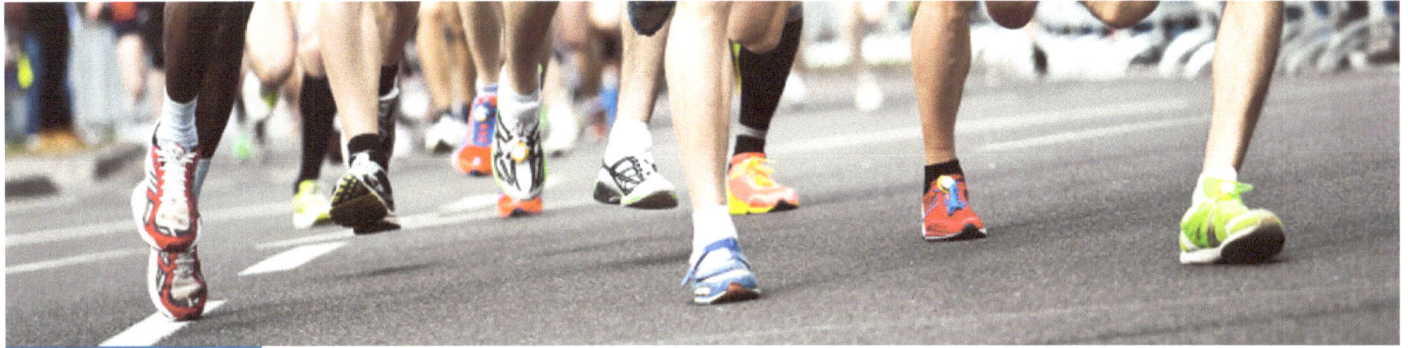

run faster, jump higher, and become stronger. Fitness centers and health clubs were popping up in every city, and existing sports clubs, tennis clubs, and athletic clubs were converting wasted space into areas with equipment where people could come to exercise.

The link between exercise and improved cardiovascular health is not a new revelation. (You can go back to ancient physicians and philosophers like Hippocrates and Siddhartha who said exercise is good for you, but they didn't have any data.) It had been over 31 years since a British doctor named Jeremy Morris completed a ground-breaking study in 1953 that showed that London bus conductors were far less likely to suffer from heart attacks than their bus driving peers. The simple act of moving up and down the double-decker steps each day made the conduc-tors less prone to heart disease.

Dr. Kenneth Cooper, founder of the Cooper Institute For Aerobics Research, had just previously come out with his renowned book "Aerobics", which outlined the guidelines for safe and proper cardiovascular benefit that is still used as a standard today.

These guidelines are:

- Figure Out Your Maximum Heart Rate (for the average person, 220 minus your age)

- Figure Out Your Safe Training Range (exercise at 70% to 85% of your maximum heart rate)

- Train Within That Range For At Least 30 Minutes

With monitoring tools such as a heart monitor, you can adjust your maximum heart rate to meet your conditioning level. Your maximum heart rate changes to some extent in relation to your fitness. This adjusted maximum heart rate is based on resting heart rate, heart rate variability at rest, age, gender, height, body weight, and maximal oxygen uptake (VO2max). All the organs involved, including the heart, lungs, muscles, and blood vessels, learn to work more efficiently.

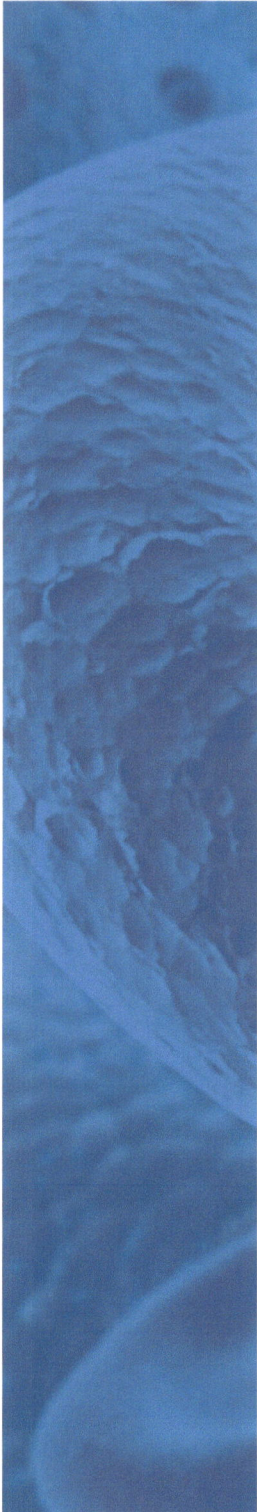

What actually happens to the body's functioning through regular aerobic exercise is a "Training Effect" in the cells. The body becomes more efficient in extracting oxygen from the blood. All the organs involved, including those previously mentioned, learn to work more effectively with less effort. This training enables the muscle fibers to become better able at obtaining oxygen from the hemoglobin in red blood cells. The lungs can take in and expel a greater volume of air in a single breath; hence, exertion produces less huffing and puffing. As this training effect progresses with regularity, the heart becomes accustomed to pumping more blood in a single stroke. The heart, with this increased stroke volume, is able to accomplish the same workload with fewer beats per minute. These two effects of training explain why athletes have slower resting heart rates and why their pulse rate returns to resting rate more quickly after exertion.

In 1984, Dr. Ralph S. Paffenbarger Jr., a researcher at the Stamford School of Medicine, published his landmark study that substantiated the link between exercise and longevity, and helped lay the foundation for the modern fitness movement. He proved that physical activity could prevent heart disease. In 1960, he launched the College Alumni Health Study, which tracked the exercise habits of 52,000 men who had entered Harvard University and the University Of Pennsylvania between 1916 and 1950 as they moved through middle and old age. Those who exercised vigorously, expending 2,000 calories a week — the equivalent of jogging or walking briskly for 20 miles — lived longer than those who didn't, the study concluded in 1986. That study took decades to complete and led to several landmark publications debunking the idea that people with a family history of heart disease who exercised could not reduce their risk. The research also showed that those who actively engaged in sports had a lower risk of death from heart disease and other illnesses associated with aging. The exercisers had death rates a quarter to a third lower than those in the study who were least active. Also, men who take up exercise later in life appeared to receive the same benefits as lifelong exercisers. (In other words it is not too late to have your cells be fit. Lack of fitness and poor health is reversible.) He showed that sedentary people are much more at risk, and the more they exercise, the better. His work influenced the 1996 Surgeon General's Report on Physical Activity and Health, as

14

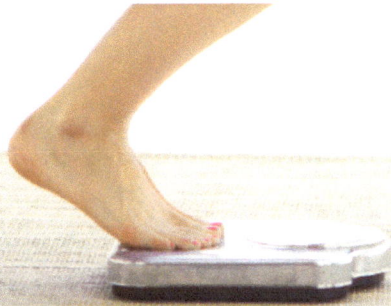

well as exercise guidelines issued by the American College of Sports Medicine and the Center For Disease Control And Prevention. There's not much more convincing people need.

[As a special note: This study was done on men. Expending calories is weight related but not gender specific. A 120 lb. woman would have to exercise longer than a 200 lb. man to expend 2,000 calories. As a result, one would conclude that a smaller person would have to expend fewer calories to get the same benefit. A simple way to calculate what your calorie output should be per week is to run or walk 4 miles, measure your calorie output, and multiply that by 5. (Walking or Running 4 miles, as you know, expends the same number of calories… it would just take longer if you walked.)]

Since 1984, continued research has proved that exercising 2,000 calories per week prevents not only heart disease but also kidney disease, stroke, diabetes, osteoporosis, cancer (colon, breast, uterine, lung, reproductive-system, lymphoma, leukemia, melanoma, Hodgkins's disease, thyroid, mouth, bladder, and eye). It also lowers blood pressure, boosts the immune system and Natural Killer Cells (NK cells), relieves symptoms of depression, controls weight, reduces risk of falling, improves lung capacity, lowers resting heart rate, improves circulation, maintains bone strength, improves lean body tissue, lowers blood sugar, improves reaction time, improves balance, reduces stress, stimulates production of human growth hormone (HGH), improves posture, and reduces accidents, just to mention a few.

For Optimal Health Your Exercise Must Be Intense Enough To Change "Bad" Cytokines To "Good" Cytokines

In 2004, Chris Crowley and Dr. Henry Lodge published a book called "Younger Next Year" that described the explosion of scientific information on how our bodies work on the cellular level. In biology there are only two things that happen… growth or decay. If a person's cells are not growing, then they are decaying. Growth is displayed by a strong, lean, fit, happy, optimistic, energetic person free of disease that lives a long time. Decay is obvious by an overweight, weak, unhappy, tired person suffering from numerous ailments and diseases. As it turns out, unfortunately for the lazy,

15

the thing that signals growth is exercise. The resounding message: you have to exercise all the time because that is who you are. For the most part, we perceive ourselves as being separate from nature. To a certain extent this is true. When man evolved the ability to stand up and walk out of nature, however, he brought with him biological systems that had been developing for millions of years. Without input from the modern world, your body will misinterpret signals and react as if it were back in nature in the early days of evolution. This is the critical factor proving why dieting alone does not work. Your body misinterprets your intention to lose weight, instead it anticipates it as if winter or a deadly peril, and signals to your body's systems that there is a need to conserve energy. The more you diet, the stronger the urge to survive, and the harder it becomes to lose the weight.

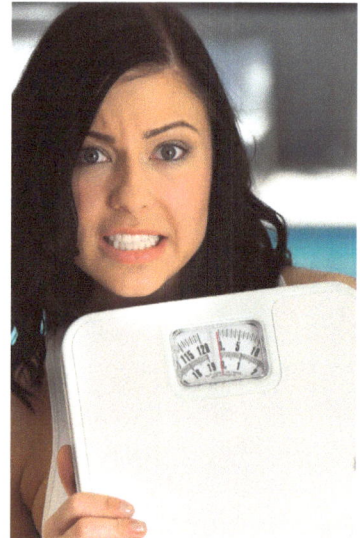

The opposite is also true. Consuming endless calories and being sedentary without exercise signals your body's systems that you're heading into a famine and that you may well not survive. You see that no matter how much food there was in one day, it spoiled and was gone the next. Man always had to get up and hunt for hours every day. So no matter how much was consumed in one day, the only reason not to get up and hunt was famine. In response, your body and brain go into a form of depression to conserve resources and slow down metabolism. They shut down for survival by letting all but the most critical systems atrophy and decay. Every day that you don't get up and move physically you're telling your body that it is time to decay, to store every scrap of excess food as fat for energy, dump the immune system, melt off the muscle, and let the joints deteriorate.

This is where the new ground-breaking science comes in. We now know that these signals come from messenger proteins in the cells called cytokines that control this process, and it happens in the cells continuously. You send billions of internal signals all day, every day. A very oversimplified description of it would be that "bad cytokines" encourage decay; "good cytokines" encourage growth. Please keep in mind that this process of conserving energy and developing diseases is not aging. What most people perceive as normal aging isn't normal. Seventy percent of all serious illness is preventable through calorie expenditure. Exercise maintains healthy systems and signals and prevents premature aging and death that are lifestyle-related. Living a full and healthy life through your 100's and beyond with vim, vigor, and vitality is a reality. Living through your 80's, bedridden, with tubes in your nose, will be your choice.

Exercise Has To Be Intense Enough To Stimulate The Proliferation Of Immune System NK Cells That Prevent Cancer

There's also good evidence that exercise can help prevent some forms of cancer. Paffenbarger's original investigation with the Harvard alumni was one of the first studies to link exercise with fewer malignancies. He showed that individuals who burned more than 2,000 calories a week had a lower cancer death rate than those who expended fewer than 500 weekly calories.

In recent years, the news about cancer and exercise have generally been positive. As an example, a new University of Southern California study indicates that women who exercise several times a week have a significantly lower risk of breast cancer than those who don't exercise. The study was conducted with over 1,000 women as subjects. It showed that females who exercise from just one to three hours per week reduce their breast cancer risk by 30 percent, while women who work out four or more hours a week lower their breast cancer chances by 50 percent! About 1 in 10 women develop it, and the disease claims about 50,000 lives a year in the United States alone. The Southern California study suggests that a large number of activities probably have equally protective effects against breast tumors. Running, cycling, swimming, soccer, aerobics, vigorous walking, and a variety of other sports were shown to deter breast cancer.

It's likely that exercise may limit the risk of other kinds of cancer as well. Moderate exercise tends to activate your immune system and can temporarily boost the activity of a unique immune-system cell - the NK

17

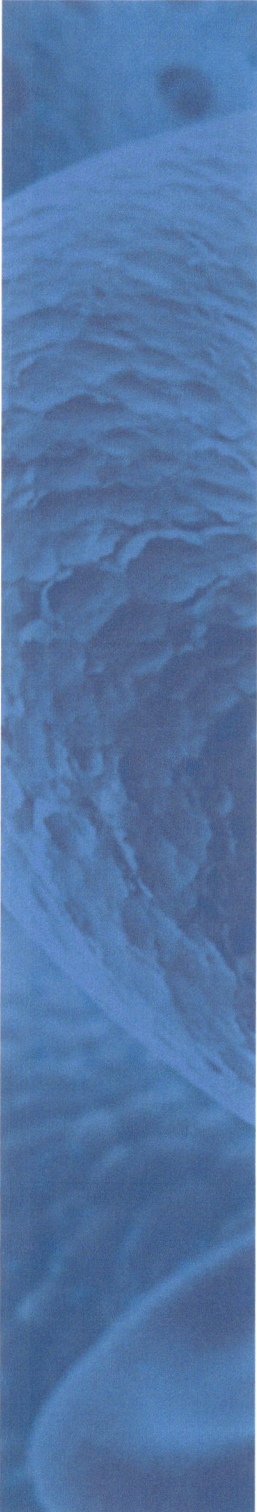

cell. Since one of the NK cells' chief duties within our body is to destroy cancer cells before they can develop into full-blown tumors, regular exercise may offer some generalized protection against cancer.

It's a good bet that intense exercise can lower the risk of lung cancer. In recent research completed at Harvard, 17,775 men were studied over a 28-year period between 1962 and 1990. The activity levels of the men were assessed using mailed questionnaires, and the subjects were classified as either inactive (expending fewer than 1,000 calories a week during exercise), moderately active (burning between 1,000-2,500 calories per week, which is the equivalent of running 10-25 miles per week), or highly active (expending more than 2,500 calories weekly during exercise). Factors which tend to increase the risk of lung cancer - smoking, age and body mass - were controlled statistically. A total of 354 lung cancers actually occurred during the research, but analysis of the data revealed that physical activity was linked with an appreciably lower risk of lung malignancy, especially in the men who were highly active throughout the 28-year study. This latter group had only half the risk of lung cancer compared to inactive males. Lung cancer accounts for about 20-25 per cent of all cancer deaths, and kills 100,000 men in the United States each year.

In addition, a number of studies have shown that exercise can reduce the risk of colon cancer. It's possible that exercise does this by helping to move materials through the intestines more quickly. Such quicker movements might flush bile acids and other potential carcinogens out of the digestive system before they can transform normal colon cells into malignancies. Preliminary research has also suggested that women who burn between 1,500 – 2,000 calories a week during exercise have lower rates of reproductive-system cancer, lymphoma, leukemia, myeloma, Hodgkin's disease, thyroid cancer, and cancers of the bladder, eye, and mouth compared to sedentary women. That's a huge chunk of disease prevention - and all for working intensively for ½ hour per day (doesn't include the time it takes to warm up or cool down, ladies).

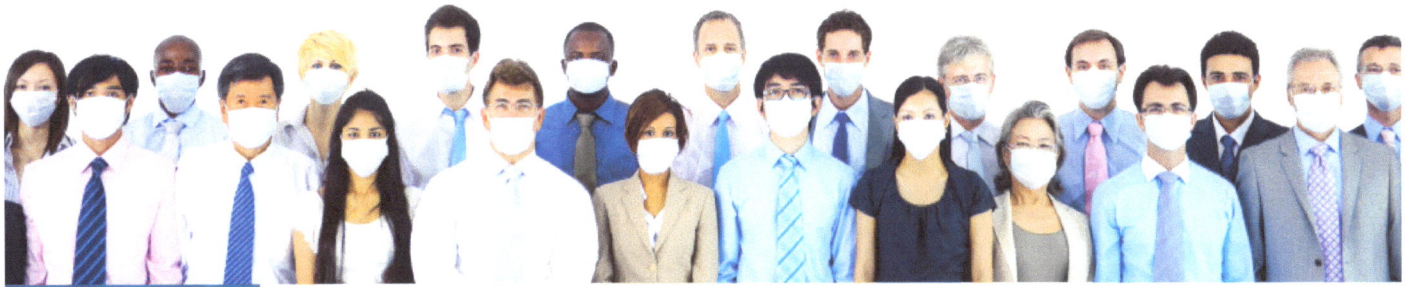

To Prevent Diabetes, Exercise Has To Be Intense Enough To Deplete Glycogen Stores To Stimulate Insulin Sensitivity

When you hear the word epidemic, you may likely think of diseases that plague thousands of people in less developed countries. However, epidemics are not exclusive to such places. In fact, the world's most widespread epidemics strike a lot closer to home than you may think. An epidemic is defined as a disease that has come to affect a large portion of a given population. The exact parameters differ among experts, but a good estimation puts the number at around 3% of a population. If the number of people affected by the disease reaches this number, it can be considered an epidemic.

Diabetes is now considered a global epidemic that is affecting not just a select number of countries but all populations. It joins a short, but unfortunately, growing list of diseases which HIV/AIDS is part of. Projections for diabetes spreading are alarming. The World Health Organization (WHO) had pegged the number of diabetes patients to reach 240 million people worldwide by the year 2010. By the end of 2011, the estimated number of diabetics would be at 285 million. Actually, the number is closer to 347 million, which is markedly higher than previous projections. Of the 347 million people with diabetes, 138 million live in China and India and another 36 million in the United States and Russia.

The disease comes in two forms: Type I (5% of cases) and Type II (90-95% of cases). Both, however, are similar in that both types involve the hormone insulin in the body and its ability to process sugar in the bloodstream. Too much or too little sugar in the body has adverse effects ranging from kidney failure, eyesight loss, and in extreme cases, coma. Type I diabetes occurs when the immune system, misled into thinking that these insulin-forming cells are harmful, attacks them (the immune system fails to recognize the cells as "self" and see them as "non-self"). The pancreas, therefore, fails to produce insulin leading to a heightened level of sugar in the body, which stresses the kidneys, and leads to further complications. Most of the patients demonstrate the disease's symptoms at around 15 years of age although the disease may have already been active years before. It is because of this that experts have interchanged the term Type I diabetes with "juvenile onset diabetes." Recently, however, this practice has been set aside in light of the alarmingly increasing number of young people contracting Type II diabetes. Type II diabetes (also known as "adult onset diabetes") is characterized by the body's failure to process sugar in the bloodstream despite the fact that insulin is produced by the pancreas. Not enough insulin is produced, or insulin sensitivity is reduced, and that the body simply cannot respond. This form of diabetes accounts for 90 percent of the estimated 300 million cases of the disease worldwide.

There is a huge correlation between Type II diabetes and obesity. Most obese individuals lead a sedentary lifestyle while consuming food high in carbohydrates, sugars, and fat. These poor eating habits, coupled with the lack of physical activity, increase the volume of sugar in the bloodstream. The pancreas cannot produce enough insulin to meet the demands of processing so much sugar and therefore diabetes sets in. If left unchecked, the complications arising from diabetes are many and adverse. Retinopathy is the degeneration of the retina of the eye, leading to loss of sight. Kidney disease, and failure sets in when the organ finally breaks down due to the excessive stress from filtering too much sugar in the blood. Nervous system disorders are experienced by around half of diabetes sufferers. Symptoms such as impaired sensation in the limbs, carpal tunnel syndrome, and even impotence, have been recorded among diabetics. When sensation is impaired in the limbs, infection from injuries may progress without being noticed, leading to no other resort but amputation. Diabetic coma (diabetic ketoacidosis) occurs when a patient becomes severely dehydrated and metabolism is greatly imbalanced. Since the cells in the body are starved of energy, the entire body shuts down, leading to a coma. These complications, however, pale in comparison to the number of lives that are lost every year due to diabetes. As of now, the number of deaths related to the disease is placed at around 4 million annually.

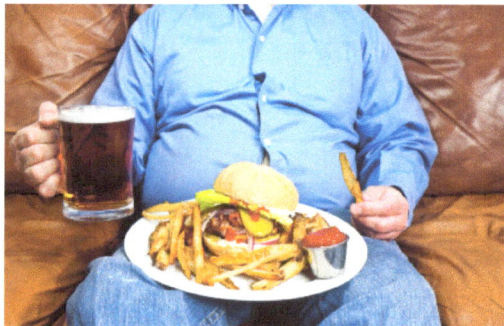

The good news… 9 cases in 10 can be avoided by taking several simple steps

Perhaps the greater tragedy is that the adverse effect of diabetes (particularly Type II) can be prevented. The good news… 9 cases in 10 can be avoided by taking several simple steps: keeping weight under control, exercising intensely enough to deplete the glycogen stores in the cells, eating a healthy diet, and not smoking.

Diabetes also appears to dramatically increase a person's risk of developing Alzheimer's disease or other types of dementia later in life, According to a new study conducted in Japan, which included more than 1,000 men and women over age 60, researchers found that people with diabetes were twice as likely as the other study participants to develop Alzheimer's disease within 15 years. They were also 1.75 times more likely to develop dementia.

Exercise Has To Be Intense Enough To Control Blood Levels Of Cholesterol And Triglycerides

Cholesterol is essential to the body and is used to build cell membranes, produce sex hormones, and form bile acids, which are necessary for the digestion of fats. It is essential that you have some cholesterol for optimal health; however, when blood levels are too high, some of the excess cholesterol is deposited on and in the artery walls, increasing the risk for heart disease. This cholesterol is a fat-soluble substance that is carried by special transporters in the blood called lipoproteins (fat-carrying protein). They enable fats and cholesterol to move within the water-based solution of the bloodstream. Lipoproteins are an essential part of a complex transport system that exchanges lipids (fats) to and from the liver, the intestine, and peripheral tissues where it is needed. The different types of lipoproteins are classified by the thickness of the protein shell that surrounds the cholesterol. There are five main classes of lipoproteins that have been identified, but only three have levels that are controlled by intense exercise and important in the prevention of heart disease and stroke. Those lipoproteins are: very low density lipoprotein (VLDL), a lipoprotein secreted by the liver that transports triglyceride to adipose tissue (body fat) and muscle; low-density lipoprotein (LDL), the primary transporters of cholesterol out of the liver, and high-density lipoprotein (HDL), involved in the reverse transport of cholesterol back to the liver.

21

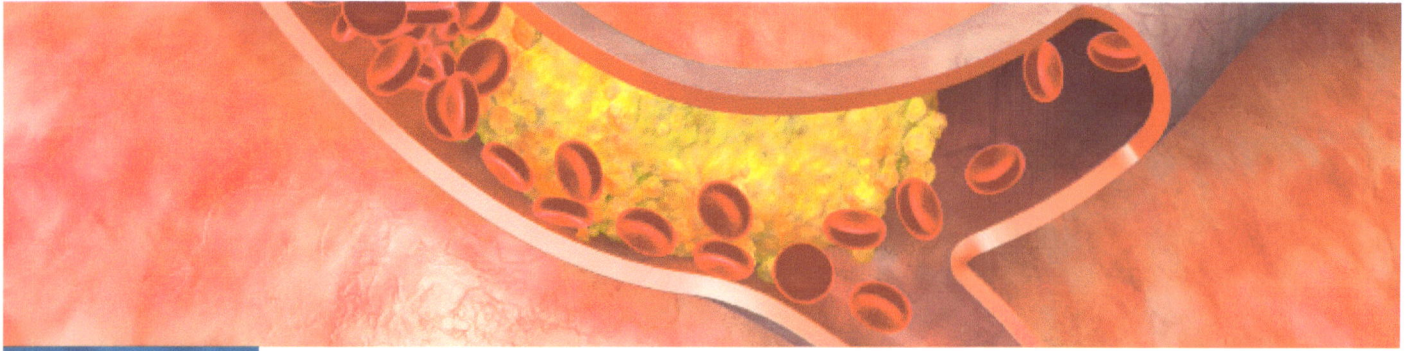

Triglycerides pound for pound contain two or three times as much energy as carbohydrates and protein. They are an efficient condensed source of energy. They come from the fats in foods (saturated and unsaturated). They are also made in the liver from carbohydrates and proteins. In the human body, high levels of triglycerides (triglycerides that have not been stored or are being used to produce energy for the human body's performance) end up in the bloodstream. They have been linked to hardening of the arteries and, by extension, the risk of heart disease and stroke. However, the relative negative impact of raised blood levels of triglycerides compared to that of LDL: HDL ratios is as yet unknown.

When a cell needs cholesterol, it makes the necessary receptors to accept the LDL-cholesterol and allows the cholesterol to enter the cell membrane. (Cholesterol is found in every cell of your body. It is especially abundant in the membranes of the cells, where it helps maintain the integrity of the membranes and plays a role in facilitating cell signaling: giving your cells the ability to communicate with each other so you function as a human, rather than just a pile of cells.) The role of LDL is to transport the fat-soluble cholesterol to various body cells through the water based blood supply. If there is an excess of LDL-cholesterol, sludge is deposited in and on the artery walls causing plaque buildup and increased risk of heart disease. LDL-cholesterol has been labeled the "bad cholesterol" because if this sludge is allowed to build up it blocks the flow of blood and also causes the arteries to harden. A desirable level of LDL is below 130 mg/dl, with an optimal level of 100 mg/dl or less. At these levels, the LDL is not deposited as sludge but is carried back to the liver.

HDL-cholesterol, sometimes called the "good" or "healthy" cholesterol, is responsible for the transport of excess cholesterol from the blood and artery walls to the liver where it is converted to bile to be used for digestion or disposed of by the body. This "reverse cholesterol transport process" is believed to be helpful in preventing or reversing heart disease. When HDL levels are above 60 mg/dl, the risk of heart disease is decreased. It is considered undesirable for HDL levels to decrease below 40 mg/dl.

A little exercise is better than none, but more is better than a little

Exercise controls optimal levels of blood cholesterol. One way is by helping you lose — or maintain — weight. Being overweight tends to increase the amount of low-density lipoprotein (LDL) in your blood.

Researchers now believe there are several mechanisms involved. First, exercise stimulates enzymes that help move LDL from the blood (and blood-vessel walls) to the liver. From there, the cholesterol is converted into bile (for digestion) or excreted. So the more you exercise, the more LDL your body expels. Second, in the November 5, 2002 issue of the New England Journal of Medicine, researchers from Duke University report that exercise produces favorable changes in lipid profiles. Exercise increases the size of the protein particles that carry cholesterol through the blood. Some of those particles are small and dense; some are big and fluffy. "The small, dense particles are more dangerous than the big, fluffy ones because the smaller ones can squeeze into the linings of the heart and blood vessels and go to work there. Now it appears that exercise increases the size of the protein particles that carry both good and bad lipoproteins."

"A little exercise is better than none, but more is better than a little"

That Duke University Medical Center study also found that more intense exercise is actually better than moderate exercise for lowering cholesterol.

In a study of overweight, sedentary people who did not change their diet, the researchers found that those who got moderate exercise (the equivalent of 12 miles of walking per week) did lower their LDL level somewhat. But the people who did more vigorous exercise (the equivalent of 20 miles of running a week) lowered it even more. Indications are that there may be a dose-response relationship between exercise and HDL levels.

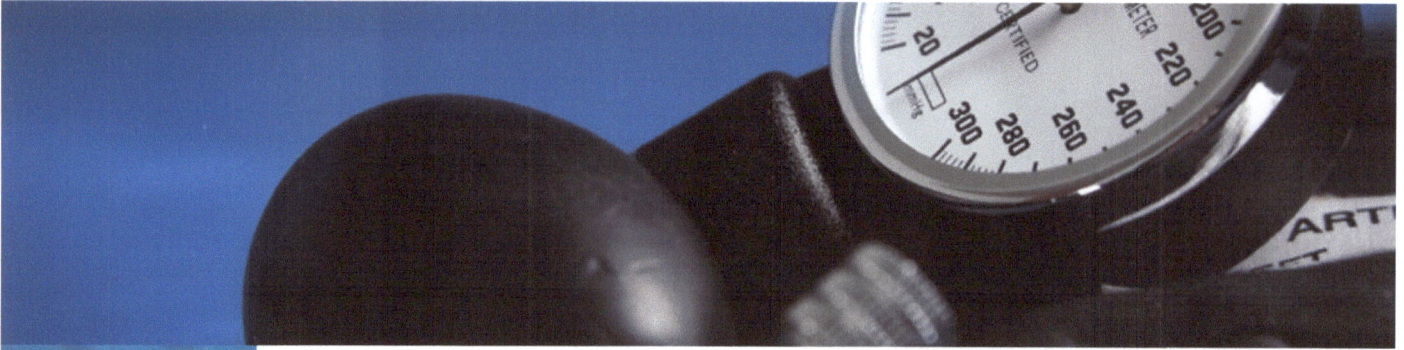

Exercise Has To Be Intense Enough To Lower Blood Pressure

Can exercise also help to control blood pressure in people with mild to moderate hypertension (high blood pressure) too? This is an important question, since high blood pressure is common in Britain and the United States. In fact, an estimated 1 in 4 adults in the US suffers from hypertension, and half of them (about 30 million people) aren't aware that they actually have the condition. Untreated hypertension can dramatically increase the risk of stroke and congestive heart failure. The available evidence suggests that exercise can reduce the risk of developing high blood pressure - and in some cases can bring down pressure in people with mild to moderate hypertension. In a recent study which followed blood pressure over time in a group of 30 hypertensive women, pressure dropped significantly when the women maintained a regular exercise program, only to rise again when exercise ceased. Investigators at the famous Cooper Clinic in Dallas, Texas, have also been able to show that individuals with low levels of fitness have a 50 percent greater risk of developing high blood pressure than those who exercise regularly. Again, such studies suggest that you don't have to be a serious athlete to have good blood pressure: regular, intense exercise will do just fine.

Why does the exercising person tend to have lower blood pressure? First, well-trained muscles usually have many more capillaries (small blood vessels) than untrained muscles. These capillaries drain off blood from the arteries, lowering overall pressure. The veins of fit people also tend to have greater capacities, again preventing pressure from building up in arteries.

Exercise can prevent high blood pressure indirectly by reducing the risk of obesity and insulin resistance, both of which increase one's chances of hypertension. Exercise has also been strongly linked with reductions in stress, which may help to keep blood pressure at moderate levels.

*One pound of fat is
equal to 3500 calories*

Exercise Has To Be Intense Enough To Reduce The % Of Body Fat

Most of us know that we need to keep excess body fat off our bodies. Understanding what is involved is important in keeping it real in reaching that objective. 1 lb. of fat is equal to 3,500 calories. In order to lose that 1 pound you must either expend 3,500 calories, cut 3,500 calories off of what you eat or a combination of exercising and cutting calories. To just diet and lose that 1lb of fat, you would have to cut 500 calories a day off of what you normally eat to maintain your body weight each day for 1 week (7 x 500 = 3,500). We have already learned that cutting calories sends signals to our body to conserve energy and to force a famine response. If you were to just exercise and expend 500 calories per day, you would lose just 1 lb. of fat each week. With most aerobic programs, weight lifting, running, or cycling you would have to exercise for 1 hour or more a day every day 7 days a week. That is probably too difficult to maintain over a long period of time. And you would only lose 1 lb. each week! A comprehensive program of both lowering and expending calories makes a lot more sense and sends the right signals that all is well. In considering what is possible and practical, a 1 to 2 lb. weight loss per week is manageable. With weight loss of more than 1 to 2 lbs. per week you start to lose muscle. It becomes counter productive and may

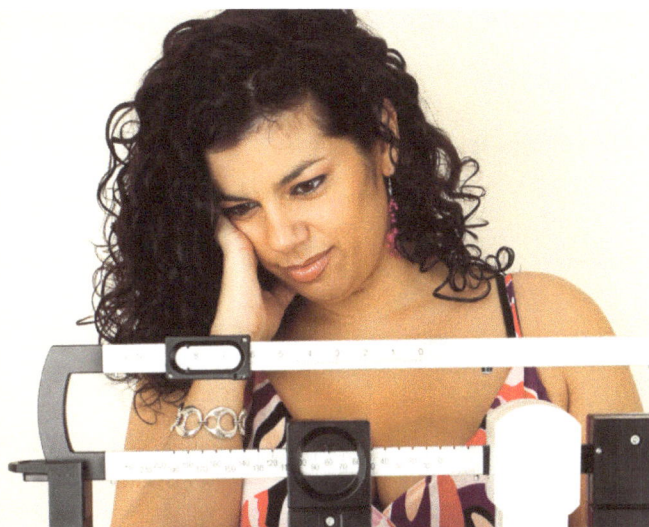

25

"When you lose weight you don't lose fat cells… they just shrink"

even be hazardous. One reason many dieters become discouraged is that the body's metabolism usually slows down in reaction to calorie restriction; exercise can help counteract that decrease. Remember: it's the signals in the cells that cause growth or decay. You want to continue to send the correct "grow signals". At the same time, regular exercise helps control appetite, making it easier to stick to a program of calorie restriction. Improved muscle tone contributes to a trimmer, healthier look, enhancing the effect of weight loss. Losing weight can also help lower your LDL (bad cholesterol) and total cholesterol levels, as well as increase HDL cholesterol (good cholesterol).

[Special note: ONE CAN NEVER LOSE FAT CELLS! An increase in the number of fat cells is called hyperplasia. It naturally happens at certain times such as late childhood and early puberty. From the five to six billion fat cells that you had when you were a baby, the number increases during childhood and puberty. During adulthood, you'll have 25 to 30 billion of these cells (with a normal body composition). Some hormonal changes result in increased metabolism, like pregnancy, and there is a tendency for these cells to increase in number. If you are overweight, your fat cells are in the range of 75 billion. If you become obese, that number increases three times - between 250 and 300 billion. The one factor that you have control over to keep those fat cells from increasing in number is your caloric intake. You get calories from what you eat… the more sugar, fats, and carbohydrates in your diet, the higher your caloric intake, usually much more than you can burn efficiently. Even those supposedly "low-content" ingredients still add up to excess calories. Anything beyond what your body needs given your daily activities will be stored as fat, which becomes harder to lose if you have more than is necessary. More caloric intake simply means more energy stored. (Even worse, when you lose weight you don't lose the fat cells… they just shrink. One could spend months successfully losing weight, take one day off and find the weight right back on. So, do not make it harder on yourself: watch what you eat.)]

Chapter 3
Exercise Must Be Effective And Efficient In A Short Period Of Time

It really doesn't matter what kind of exercise you do as long as you meet the requirements of intense exercise. That is expending 2,000 calories per week and exercising at least 75% of your maximum heart rate. For example, walking 20 miles a week or running 20 miles a week expends the same number of calories, but walking doesn't get your heart rate up above 75%. It is better for you to walk rather than to sit and do nothing, but it doesn't meet the requirements for you to get true and complete health assurance. Running, on the other hand, meets the requirements but is counterproductive because of the stresses and pounding it puts on the body. Weight lifting and taking a long time between sets doesn't burn that many calories and doesn't raise your heart rate up high enough. Cycling and spinning classes offer a low injury risk way of exercising but are leg driven only. They offer some leg strength and leg endurance development. They are, however, linear (with no lateral movement) and leg driven only. Initially, they are a very good way to achieve aerobic benefit because they get your heart rate high enough. Because there are no lateral movements and no use of the upper torso involved in the exercise, cycling soon becomes very limited. The training effect starts to plateau, and heart rates cannot get high enough. Because cycling doesn't address the other aspects of exercise, those aspects have to be done separately. These are the normal generic subscriptions of most health clubs, fitness centers and personal trainers' programs. Separating the aspects of fitness into cardiovascular or aerobic, stretching or flexibility, core, and strength training makes exercising take too long for busy people to work into their lifestyles practically.

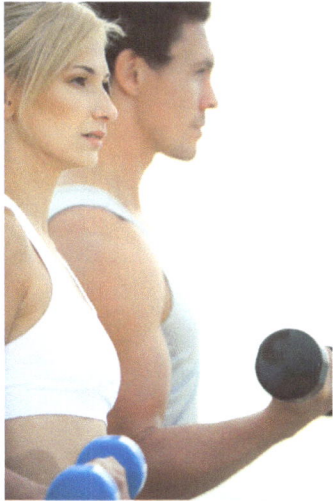

The concept of Panaerobics, developed by Dr. Leonard Schwarz, is the answer to solving this dilemma. Panaerobics maximizes and optimizes all the muscle groups of the body, not just the linear movements of the leg. You do aerobic, strength, flexibility, and strength endurance training with both linear and lateral movements all at once. It is a revolutionary fitness program that people rarely use. What you get is a higher level of fitness than that produced by any other form of aerobic exercise. It burns more calories than any other form of fitness training. It brings strength plus endurance to all of the muscles. No muscle group is neglected. Muscles already trained by other exercise and sports are even further upgraded. Intense panaerobic exercise actually feels surprisingly easy and by doing all the phases of exercise at one time it makes you burn calories like crazy. One can become as strong as most lifters, as swift as most runners, and outwork both with a smaller investment of time and with far fewer injuries. The idea is to get all the muscles of the body multitasking, if you will, to help in the conditioning of the heart. Most conventional aerobic exercise uses only the large muscles of the legs to drive the conditioning process. Instead of exercising strenuously for 4 hours per week, as in Paffenbarger's study, the same calories could be expended, (2,000 Cal), in 2 1/2 hours per week. With Panaerobics you use hand held weights to get the muscles of the upper body and torso incorporated, attaining a conditioning level far beyond conventional programs. Along with burning more calories than any other form of exercise, Panaerobics builds strength plus endurance to all of the muscles. It stretches muscles while they are warm (both dynamic and static stretching). It improves balance and proprioception. It offers efficient calorie expenditure aiding in rapid weight loss. It is safe with a very low risk of injury. It doesn't require a lot of equipment, and doesn't require a lot of space (4' x 6' area). No muscle group is neglected. And most exciting of all, the simultaneous movement of various muscles is a superlative way to train the heart and lungs. All the advantages of Panaerobics have been measured and verified with data to prove its effectiveness. In Dr. Schwartz's "Heavyhands, The Ultimate Exercise" book you will find the astonishing workloads and calorie expenditure made possible through the practice of this revolutionary program. In the book there are comparisons of other forms of exercise, their work output and caloric expenditure. Panaerobics is not only the best

The Limit Of Conditioning Level Has Not Been Approached

way for those who want to achieve the health benefits in a short period of time, but it's the only way to improve your overall fitness if you are already a world class athlete. The limit of conditioning level has not even been approached. Plateaus and increased workout times to stay at the same fitness levels are erased. Just simply increase either the amount of hand held weight or increase the cadence as your conditioning level improves. This increases the intensity and the conditioning level. The length of time needed to exercise does not have to increase for one to continue to get higher levels of conditioning and higher expenditure of calories.

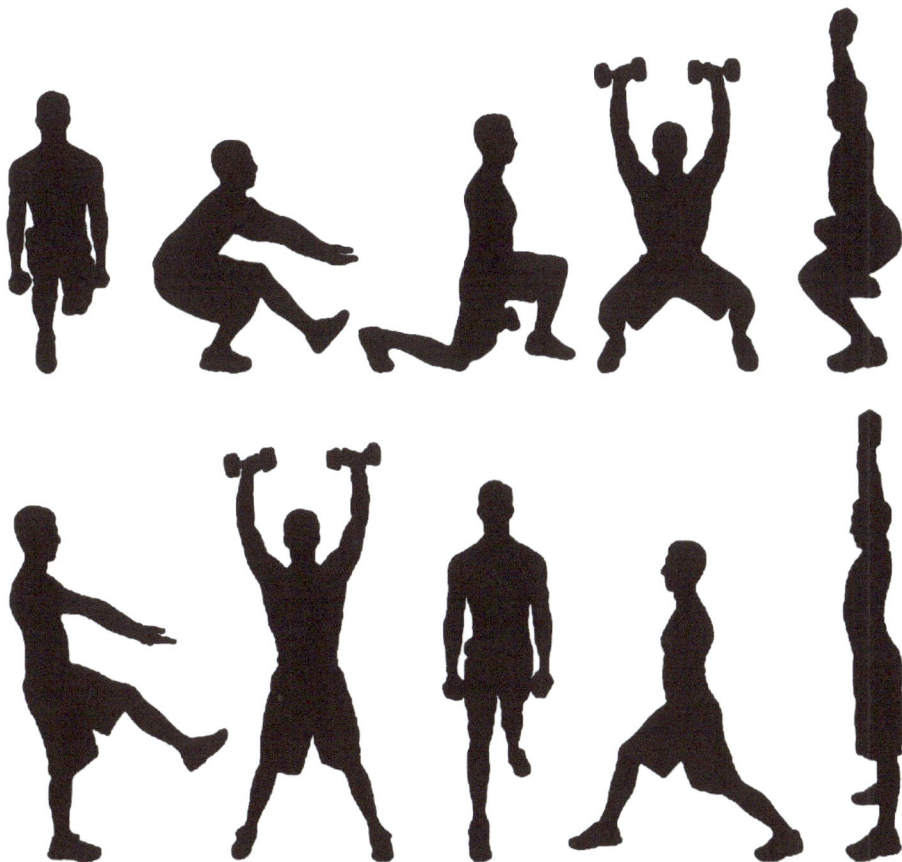

29

We live in fast-paced, high pressure, nonstop world

How To Send The Right Signals To Your Body, As If It Were Back In Nature…And Still Enjoy Living In The 21st Century

Understanding what it was like when man originated — and adapting that information to your daily life — is the key to achieving your weight loss, fitness, and health goals. We live in a fast-paced, high pressure, nonstop world, where men, women and children are on the go all the time. We live in safety and a time of plenty. We become ill because we are not connected to our roots. We have forgotten our past, and how our mind and body were made. And as a result, we contract terrible and unnecessary sicknesses. Our bodies do not know how to understand this new language, and we eat ourselves to death. We spend an enormous amount of energy living our lives with a body that was developed to live in nature. Everything you do physically, everything you eat, everything you think and feel, every emotion and experience changes your body and your brain in physical ways that were set in stone many millions of years ago. Because your body's systems are blind, the only way to fool them into believing that your body is still in nature is simply to exercise. Physical exercise triggers great waves of "grow" messages that are signaled throughout your body and mind.

Enough Exercise Is The Underlying Miracle That Prevents The Diseases Of Aging

Building on the efforts of so many who have contributed to the scientific understanding of how exercise is the underlying miracle to preventing the diseases of aging, I have designed a fitness program that I consider innovative to the health and fitness industry. It is called The Max Performance Fitness Program. It simply eliminates many of the problems traditionally faced when trying to get faster, safer, continued results from exercise.

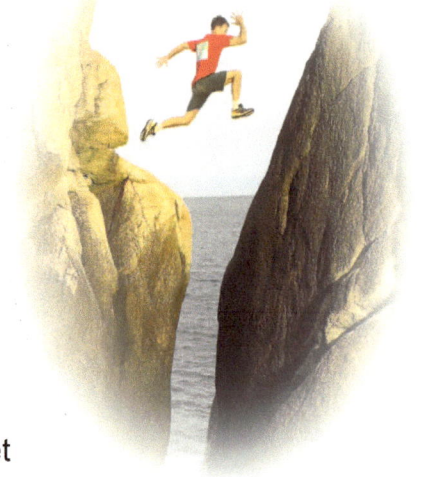

It can even eliminate 70% of all diseases and even accidents, like falls, which our society unfortunately accepts as being normal as people age. THE MAX Performance Fitness Program has an identified beginning and middle, but no end. You can do this program anywhere to get fast results without fear of getting hurt. It burns more calories than any other form of exercise in the same time period, yet doesn't take long to do. It is systematized to assure that all phases of fitness, defined by the new scientific understanding, are addressed in the shortest amount of time. It measures your progress and gives you an evaluation of your progress every 3 months. You can do it in groups or in the privacy of your own home; or you can take it with you when you travel. Finally, it clears up all the confusion of what to do and whom to listen to. It gives you the confidence to know that what you are doing will take you to where you want to go in terms of improving your health, losing weight, looking your best, and extending your life.

This program uses hand-held weights to incorporate your upper body into the exercises, and it does not rely on the legs alone to drive the conditioning process (as is often the case with running and other forms of cardio-vascular exercise). There is an emphasis on using all the muscle groups of the body, incorporating aerobic conditioning, strength, strength endurance, balance, and flexibility training, and using the muscles in their complete range of motion to get the maximum calorie expenditure from your workouts. If you're not an athlete seeking the highest levels of conditioning, you can do this in 3 1-hour workouts or 6 1/2-hour workouts weekly. The only requirement is that you burn 2,000 calories per week.

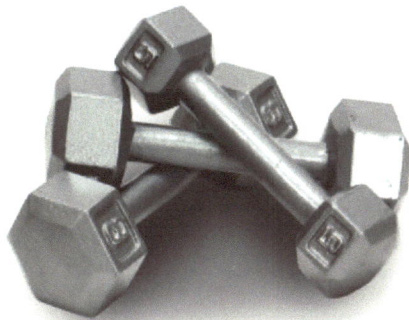

"To get results quickly you need to maximize and optimize all the muscles of your body"

Six Major Problems That You Face With Traditional Fitness Programs And How THE MAX Performance Program Overcomes Them All!

1. Results Come Too Slowly!

Traditional methods separate aerobic training, strength training, and flexibility exercises. Aerobic training is either done in classes or out on the road, running or cycling. These methods of conditioning are mostly leg-driven, but the legs are never used in their full range of motion. Once the legs have become conditioned it's very difficult to continue to get results. Compression forces are a huge problem and it's hard to prevent injuries. Strength training is done with either free weights or machines. Long rests between exercises give no aerobic benefit at all and calorie expenditure is difficult to achieve. Flexibility exercises are performed in stretch or in yoga classes. It is not realistic to believe that anyone would have enough time to do all different aspects of training separately. In order to get results quickly you need to maximize and optimize all the muscles of the body, progressively increase the intensity, and combine all the phases of exercise into a single program. This reduces the time that you must spend and increases its effectiveness. Results come immediately and there are no plateaus.

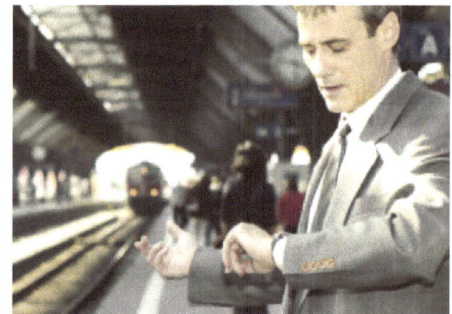

2. It Takes Too Much Time!

How do you meet all the parameters necessary to benefit from:

- Cardiovascular and aerobic conditioning
- Strength and strength endurance training
- Stretching
- Muscular definition
- Balance
- Weight control
- Calorie expenditure
- Exercise intensity

without spending enormous amounts of time doing it?

32

For every hour that a person exercises he/she gets roughly two extra hours of life

Traditional methods of training suggest that you do separate training for each of these benefits. Those workouts would take 4 to 8 hours a week. Guess What?—With THE MAX Performance Program YOU DO IT ALL AT ONCE! And it takes only 2-1/2 hours a week. Spend the time now or lose the time later. For every hour that a person exercises he/she gets roughly two extra hours of life.

3. Will I Get Hurt?

Most people believe that running is the best way to get the highest level of aerobic conditioning. The problem is that running is a leg-driven only program, and the legs are not even used in their complete range of motion. The arms are not used. This means that in order to continue to get the training effect you must run longer and faster. Another problem is that the compression forces on the ankles, knees, and hip joints are 2 to 7 times the body weight. The faster you run, the more the compression force. In the first 2 years, after initiating a running training program, over 65% of runners will have an injury that prevents them from continuing, or they will develop a nagging injury that lasts a long time.

THE MAX Performance Program is conducted in a 4' x 6' space (the size of a mat) using light weights. There is very little compression; the movements are performed at a safe pace, and in a complete range of motion. Injuries are surprisingly rare. Flexibility and balance exercises are incorporated into the movements. The exercise is intense enough that you get the aerobic benefit as well as burning a lot of calories in a short period of time. If the exercises are done at a moderate and steady pace, in their full range and at an intensity that has been proven to be safe with light weights, quick and injury-free results are guaranteed.

Most people believe that you have to use heavy weights to gain strength. People who do often develop real problems with pulled or torn muscles or tendon or ligament damage. With THE MAX Performance Program light hand-held weights are used — 10 lbs. is more than most can use. As a result, stress to muscles, joints, tendons, and ligaments is very small. Multiple and varied movements strengthen them as well.

4. The Moves I Have To Learn Are Too Difficult!

Most aerobic dance and yoga programs and weight machines are too difficult to learn, and change all the time. With THE MAX Performance Program the routines are calisthenic moves and are fairly easy to learn. If you are a beginner, the moves are modified so that you can do the program right off the bat. As you become more flexible, your heart gets into better shape, your muscles get stronger. You can begin to increase the range of motion which increases the intensity of the exercises. This program is not only the best way for those who want to achieve all of the health benefits quickly, but it's the only way to improve your overall fitness if you are already a world class athlete. The limit of conditioning has not even been approached. Plateaus and increasing exercise time to stay at the same levels are erased. Simply increase either the amount of weight or increase the cadence and continue to do the exercises completely and consistently as your conditioning level is improved. Duration need not be increased to continue to get higher and higher levels of conditioning. The exercise feels the same or easier at higher workloads.

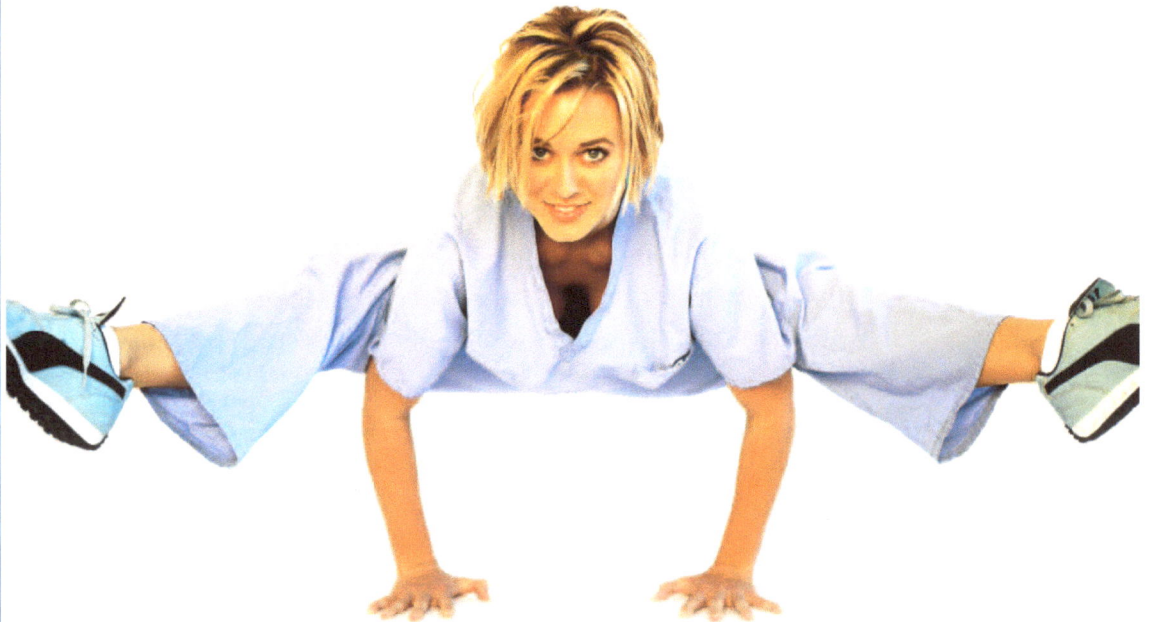

5. There Is No Way To Know How I am Doing!

With most other programs, you are left on your own after you have been given the initial instruction. You are left without an evaluation of where you started, what is the next step, and where you are going. THE MAX Performance Program has an evaluation process built into the program. Testing is part of every step you take. An initial evaluation assesses your starting level of fitness and health. Results come almost instantly, and are measured every 3 months to chart your progress. You start off without any weights to get the feel of the exercises and to work out initial stiffness. Gradually you increase weights, range of motion, flexibility, balance, aerobic capacity, strength, and strength endurance, to accommodate your fitness level and your body type.

6. I Continue To Pay For Equipment And Space That I Don't Use Or Want!

Memberships at a typical health club pay for the equipment and space. Traditionally, all aspects of training are separated into different areas of the club. For example there would be a separate area for aerobics, one for weights and weight machines, and maybe a pool. It will take you 4 to 8 hours per week to achieve the calorie expenditure to keep pace with your natural energy requirements using these traditional set-ups and programs. Rarely do fees go into designing a custom program or teaching you what you need to know — and do — to get fast, continued results. Rarely do they evaluate your progress or measure your results. THE MAX Performance Program requires very little equipment and needs only a 4'x 6' space. We evaluate your fitness and progress from the start, and you pay only for the program that you use. We highly recommend that you get a heart monitor to use during every workout to exercise at the appropriate heart rate, to keep track of calories expended, to keep your program safe, and to make sure that your exercise program is sending the right signals to your cells.

"You will prevent disease, increase quality of your life and slow the aging process"

You Can Become Younger Next Year

Changing your physical conditioning and fitness doesn't happen overnight. Changing the cellular signals does… and yes, you have to do the work and follow the program every day. Now for the first time, a concrete definition of what you have to do has been spelled out. You can prevent disease if you follow the procedures: you will increase the quality of your life and slow the aging process. You can become younger next year, and reach your personal fitness goals by assessing your current body age in relation to your chorological age, focusing on your health, and expending 2,000 calories per week. For more information on how to learn this program, to get a fitness assessment, or to get more information about weight loss, your fitness, and health, go to www.theMaxPerformance.com.

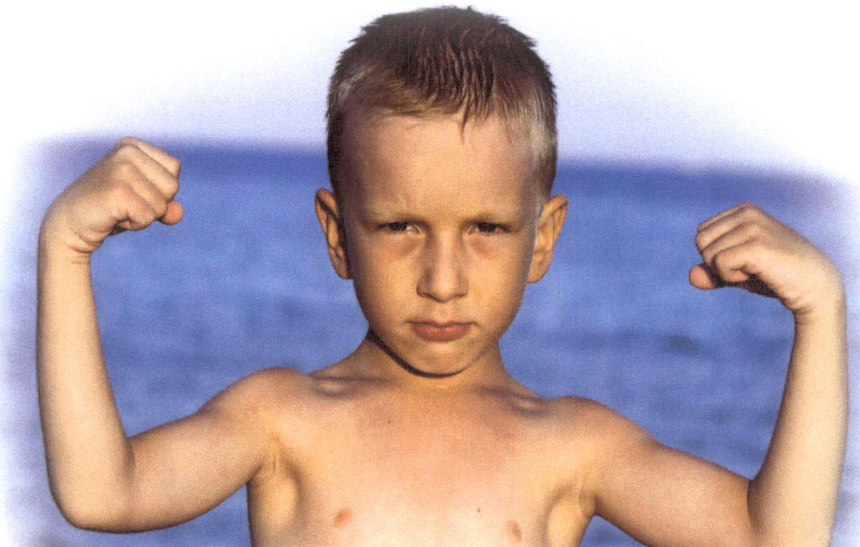

Exercise Methods Comparison Table

0 = Little Effect   10 = Maximum Effect

Exercise Method	Conditioning Aspects	0	1	2	3	4	5	6	7	8	9	10
Running	Aerobic Conditioning								▓			
	Strength Training	▓										
	Flexibility	▓										
	Strength Endurance											
	Balance			▓								
	Stress / Risk Of Injury									▓		
Weight Lifting	Aerobic Conditioning	▓										
	Strength Training											▓
	Flexibility	▓										
	Strength Endurance	▓										
	Balance	▓										
	Stress / Risk Of Injury								▓			
High Impact Aerobics	Aerobic Conditioning							▓				
	Strength Training	▓										
	Flexibility				▓							
	Strength Endurance	▓										
	Balance							▓				
	Stress / Risk Of Injury								▓			
Cycling	Aerobic Conditioning						▓					
	Strength Training			▓								
	Flexibility	▓										
	Strength Endurance			▓								
	Balance	▓										
	Stress / Risk Of Injury		▓									
Stretching	Aerobic Conditioning											
	Strength Training											
	Flexibility										▓	
	Strength Endurance											
	Balance						▓					
	Stress / Risk Of Injury				▓							
Your Exercise Program	Aerobic Conditioning											
	Strength Training											
	Flexibility											
	Strength Endurance											
	Balance											
	Stress / Risk Of Injury											
The MAX Performance FITNESS PROGRAMS	Aerobic Conditioning											▓
	Strength Training											▓
	Flexibility											▓
	Strength Endurance											▓
	Balance										▓	
	Stress / Risk Of Injury		▓									

The time that it takes to complete each aspect of conditioning = 1 hour.

The time that it takes to complete all aspects of conditioning = 3 to 5 hours.

The time exposed to high stress and risk of injury = 3 to 5 hours.

The time that it takes to complete THE MAX = 1/2 hour.

The time that it takes to complete all aspects of conditioning = 1/2 hour per day.

The time exposed to low risk of injury = 1/2 hour per day.

The extra time allowed for other things = 4 to 8 hours per week.

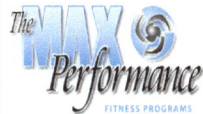

Chapter 4
Reduce Injuries, Accidents And Falls

Running has been the exercise method that many believe is the best way to get the training effect and cardiovascular conditioning. When Kenneth H. Cooper published his first bestseller, "Aerobics," in 1968, launching a worldwide fitness revolution, he was recognized as the leader of the international physical fitness movement and credited with motivating more people to exercise in pursuit of good health than any other person. In 1968, only 100,000 people were jogging in America. That number is now more than 30 million strong. Statistics show that of those 30 million folks most are already injured or will be injured from running. Initially, jogging is a very good way to achieve aerobic benefit, but soon becomes limited when the conditioning effect starts to plateau. Running is solely a leg-driven activity. The legs are the only muscles that are used to drive the conditioning process and are used only in a minimal range of motion to propel the body forward. The rest of the body's muscles aren't used. (Remember, the criteria for getting the maximum benefit from exercise are to expend 2,000 calories per week and maintaining a 75% of maximum heart rate pace for 30 minutes per day.) People have to run longer and faster to continue getting the training effect and benefits. As one starts to go faster and longer, the injuries to the feet, ankles, calves, knees, thighs, buttocks, hips, and back creep into the picture from compression forces of 2 to 7 times body weight. As a result, 65% of all exercisers and athletes who use running as a method for conditioning will have some kind of an injury within the first two years after starting a running program. Eventually, all (yes all) will suffer some kind of injury and will not be able to continue to run as a full time exercise solution.

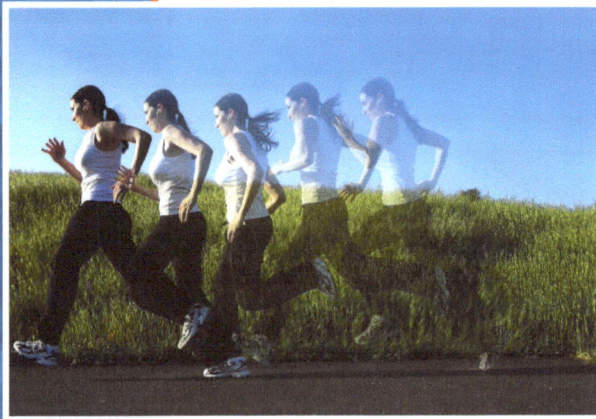

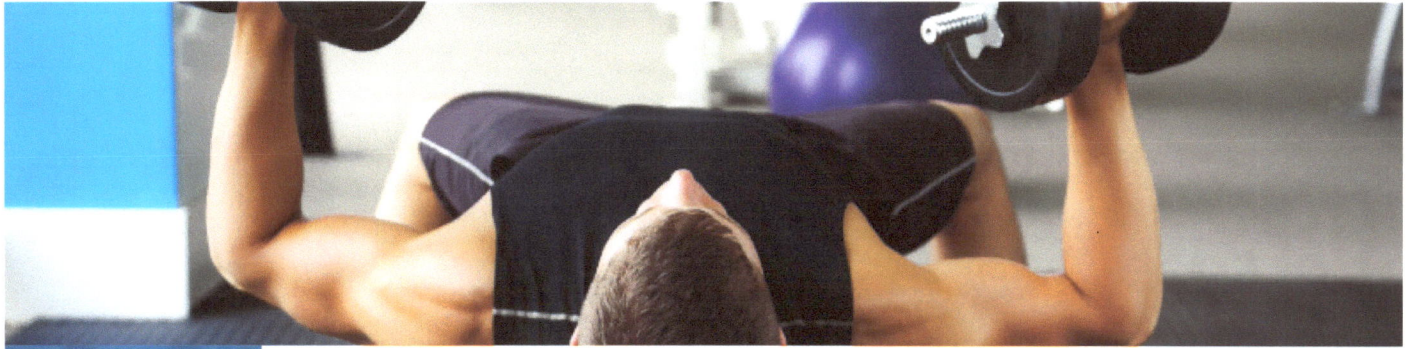

[Think of it like this: If one were to stick one's hand into a boiling pot of water, what is the percentage of people that get burned?]

Because running provides no strength, strength endurance, or flexibility training, all those activities are usually done separately. This adds more time to the process, adds more time to be subjected to potential injury and takes time away from other demands of your daily schedule. Worse yet, some that have chosen running as a way to be healthy have died from it by being exposed to dangerous situations on the roadways and have been killed by a distracted or careless driver.

[Special note: 25 % of all exercise and sports related injury are ankle injuries. Prevention of ankle injuries represents a major issue in sports medicine. Exercisers and athletes who wear Ankle Stabilizing Orthosis (ASO) nylon ankle braces were 2.6 times less likely to be injured and recovered two days sooner than exercisers with no protection or athletes who used tape. With so many injuries that occur to the ankle from exercising, recreational athletics, and sports, it would only make sense for you to wear them before you get hurt.]

Heavy weight training with free weights and machines that isolate different muscle groups is an effective way to build strength if done properly. It provides neither aerobic nor anaerobic benefit nor provides flexibility, strength endurance, or balance training. Overstressing muscles, tendons, and ligaments with sloppy form, along with holding one's breath and lifting too much weight, lead to unnecessary injuries. Health clubs and fitness areas allocate 80 percent of the square footage to strength training equipment. Fitness professionals place a tremendous emphasis on building strength and waste their clients an enormous amount of time and money trying to achieve it. Strength without endurance is pointless. Because of the time wasted and lack of development of the other essential aspects of conditioning, those aspects have to be addressed separately. This adds more time to the conditioning process and takes time away from getting the desired result when you set out to reap all the benefits of exercise.

Stretching is probably the most misunderstood aspect of exercise. Some believe that stretching is the only activity that they need to do. Most believe

"There is nothing more ridiculous than stretching cold muscles"

that they should stretch or are instructed to stretch as a warm-up and then go onto another phase of conditioning. The evidence proves that stretching before a workout is just not wise. Researchers at Temple University found that increasing the temperature of muscle fibers makes stretching more effective. They suggest warming up with light but progressively intense exercise before stretching. Only after your muscles are warm should you start to do stretching exercises to improve suppleness and flexibility. Incorporating stretching into your exercise while you do certain moves (dynamic stretching) adds additional efficiency to your stretching. Placing static stretching (stretching by holding movements and slowly increasing and holding) at the end of workouts helps you to get more range of movement. A greater range of movement also helps you burn more calories, gain more strength, and condition the cardiovascular system. This leads to faster results. If this aspect of training is conducted as a warm-up, very little benefit from it will occur. There is nothing more ridiculous than stretching cold muscles. If stretching is done as a sole activity (as in yoga or in flexibility classes), very little health benefit will come from it, and other aspects of training will either be neglected, or more time will have to be devoted to them. It has been suggested that stretching prevents injuries, and common and practical sense would dictate that this is true. There are, however, no scientific studies that I could find that indicate this is so. I would suggest that some kind of sense should take precedence here, and one should strive to develop general flexibility and that by doing so would be less prone to injury because of it.

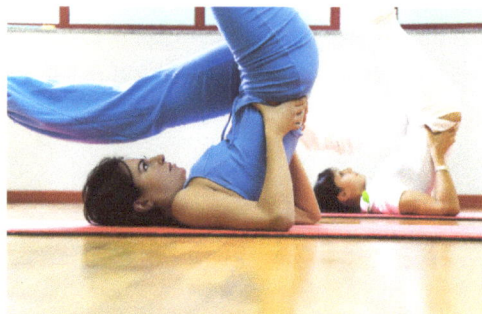

Being physically fit and healthy will go a long way in preventing accidents. You will be more alert with a better response and reaction time. You will be more flexible and see things coming from wider angles. There's also a lot of scientific evidence that exercise can reduce tension and make people less angry. The first studies in this area were conducted in the 1970s and generally showed that physically fit people were more

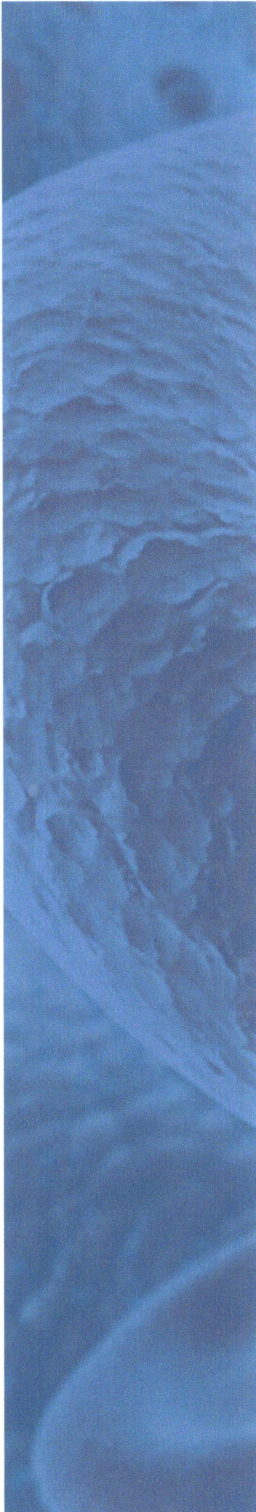

likely to report that they felt "very happy," while the less-fit more often indicated that they were "not so happy." Since then, a number of studies have shown that exercise can reduce anxiety, and "exercise therapy" has been used successfully to treat people with chronic nervousness. Some studies have actually shown that 15 minutes of exercise is better than a tranquillizer at relieving muscle tension. More than half-a-dozen separate pieces of research have shown that exercise can be helpful in the treatment of depression; these studies suggest that symptoms of depression decrease as exercise levels increase. Some psychologists have gone so far as to suggest that inactivity is itself an independent risk factor for depression. A classic piece of research completed in the 1960s revealed that individuals who exercised regularly exhibited more humor, optimism, ambition, patience, and energy than did non-exercisers. The study also found that regular exercisers were more easy-going and good-tempered. Follow-up studies asserted that regular exercisers were more imaginative and had more self-assurance and emotional stability than sedentary individuals. Such surveys have often been criticized on the ground that happy, confident people might simply be more likely to decide to exercise than unhappy ones - in other words, that exercise might be an outcome, not a cause, of happiness. However, subsequent research has shown that exercise programs can indeed produce gains in self-confidence, emotional stability and self-sufficiency, and that exercise can also increase overall vigor, and reduce fatigue and tension. All this can be attributed to preventing accidents.

How does exercise produce all these important psychological effects? Scientists at Oregon Health and Science University in 2003 showed that exercise can actually change the concentrations of neurotransmitters - chemicals that nerve cells use to communicate with each other - in the brain. Exercise can dramatically increase the levels of a group of chemicals called the endorphins. They reduce sensations of pain and tend to induce a sense of tranquility. Happily enough, you don't have to exercise for very long to get an endorphin "rush": studies suggest that just 30 minutes of vigorous activity is often enough to bathe your brain cells in these chemicals. Research has shown that those who exercise regularly are less "stressed out" by unpleasant events like exposure to

"There's even evidence that exercise can make you smarter"

loud noises or cold temperatures. This resistance to stress seems to be particularly pronounced during approximately a six-hour period which follows every workout. Exercisers also seem better able to cope with life's major negative events, such as divorce, the death of a loved one, or a large financial loss. It's not that exercisers are not bothered by such events. Instead, they seem less debilitated and more able to reconstruct their lives following an emotionally damaging experience.

There's even evidence that exercise can make you smarter. A study published in the Journal of Neuroscience confirmed that exercise increases the chemical BDNF - brain-derived neurotrophic factor - in the hippocampus, a curved, elongated ridge in the brain that controls learning and memory. BDNF is involved in protecting and producing neurons in the hippocampus.

Individuals who exercise throughout life seem to have better memory retention as they get older, and studies have also shown that people who exercise often simultaneously improve their mathematical and reasoning abilities.

Getting back to the physical benefits of exercise, we know that regular exercise can strengthen your skeletal system, reducing your chances of developing osteoporosis, a bone-thinning disease that affects about one out of every two women and one out of five men during their lifetimes. This, along with strengthening the muscles and training balance, helps prevent falls, which have proven many times to be a fatal.

There's even evidence to suggest that regular exercise can lower your risk of coming down with the common cold. Various studies indicate that individuals who exercise from about one to three hours a week have a reduced risk of upper respiratory infection, compared to individuals who exert themselves for less than that.

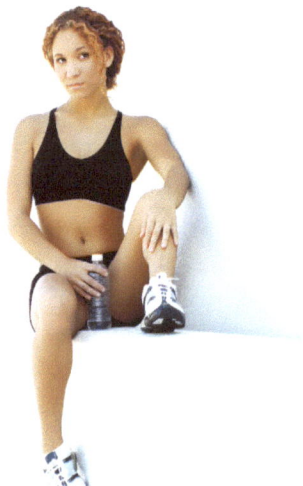

42

Chapter 5
Measure Results

It has been my experience that people get crazy over their measurements. Now I know you wouldn't do this, but many people have a false sense or perception of their measurements. For example, I had a buddy of mine get so angry with me that we almost got into a fist fight. I laughed when he indicated that his waist measurement was 36 inches. He had just purchased a new waist size 36 jeans and obvious to me that measurement was below his 46 inch measurement at his belly button. It is important that we do not become seduced by our daily experience and perceptions into false beliefs about the true nature of things. Remember figures never lie. But liars always figure. Don't shoot the messenger by slamming the scale, throwing the tape measure across the room, or punching somebody out. Take the measurements and see them for what they are, which is the true indication of your compliance to what you have set your goals to be.

Measure Your Body Mass Index (BMI)

I would have to say, and it is just an observation I make without measuring it, that most professional Baseball players and American Football players are overweight according to BMI measurements and some are just downright obese.

Body Mass Index (BMI) is a number calculated from a person's weight and height. BMI is a fairly reliable indicator of body fatness for most people. BMI does not measure body fat directly, but research has shown that BMI correlates to direct measures of body fat, such as underwater weighing and dual-energy x-ray absorptiometry (DXA). BMI can be considered an alternative for direct measures of body fat. Additionally, BMI is an inexpensive and easy-to-perform method of screening for weight categories that may lead to health problems. In order to calculate your body mass index, simply Google BMI and click on any one of the calculators. Then put your height and weight in the appropriate place, and the score is calculated.

Score of:

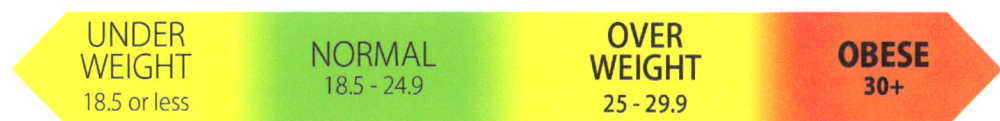

UNDER WEIGHT
18.5 or less

NORMAL
18.5 - 24.9

OVER WEIGHT
25 - 29.9

OBESE
30+

There are three ways to measure your cholesterol levels

Measure Your Calorie Expenditure And Heart Rate While Exercising

In order for people to have any idea how many calories they are expending, they have to measure calorie expenditure during their workout. One way is to use a heart monitor that includes calorie expenditure as one of its readouts and is worn during exercise. If you are guessing at how many calories you are expending during workouts, I guarantee you are not expending enough. Along with the calorie output, the right heart monitor will tell you if you are working out in a safe heart-rate range and will tell you if your workout is intense enough. Get a heart monitor that has the capability to measure your fitness with a fitness test. Your maximum heart rate changes to some extent in relation to your fitness. This adjusted maximum heart rate is based on resting heart rate, heart rate variability at rest, age, gender, height, body weight, and maximal oxygen uptake (VO2max). This fitness test measures your aerobic/cardiovascular fitness at rest and will predict your maximal oxygen uptake (VO2max) in just five minutes. VO2 max is the maximum volume of oxygen that the body can consume during intense whole-body exercise while breathing air at sea level. This volume is expressed as a rate of liters per minute (L/min). Because oxygen consumption is linearly related to energy expenditure, when we measure oxygen consumption, we are indirectly measuring an individual's maximal capacity to do work aerobically. That capacity will increase as one increases one's fitness level.

Measure Your Blood Cholesterol Levels

There are three ways to evaluate cholesterol score, which are often used in concert with each other. Measurements typically taken to determine cholesterol score include total cholesterol, and individual cholesterol measurements for high-density lipoproteins (HDL) and low-density lipoproteins (LDL). When these measurements are read together, the doctor has the best way of determining your cholesterol score and cholesterol health. Testing may also include an evaluation of triglyceride level.

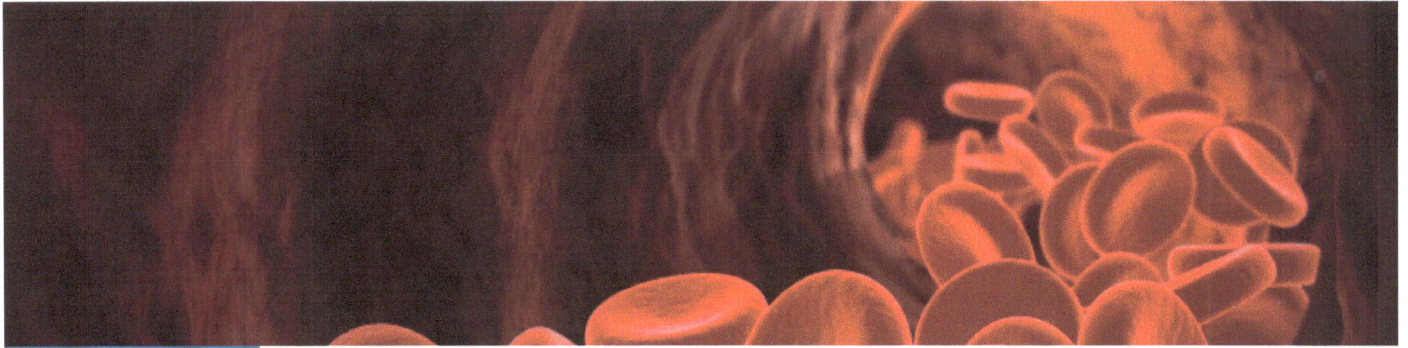

When evaluating total cholesterol level, the desired cholesterol score should be less than 200 milligrams per deciliter (mg/dL). A score between 200-239 mg/dL is considered borderline high and a score of 240 mg/dL or above is high. Many physicians suggest patients try to aim for a cholesterol level of about 150-180 mg/dL by modifying diet and pursuing exercise. When this is accomplished, the total cholesterol score is considered safe.

LDL measurements tend to measure the "bad" cholesterol, which is most likely to lead to disease. So, in this case you are looking for a low number. A good cholesterol score of LDL is between 100-129 mg/dL. A score under 100 mg/dL is considered optimal. An LDL cholesterol score of 130-159 mg/dL is borderline high, 160-189 mg/dL is high, and 190 mg/dL is very high. With the LDL measurement and the total cholesterol measurement, you want to see these numbers lower instead of higher.

In contrast, HDL cholesterol score is better when the number is higher. This is the "good cholesterol" our body needs — it keeps total cholesterol and LDL numbers down. A good cholesterol score for HDL is 60 mg/dL or better. 40 mg/dL or lower is considered a risk factor for developing heart disease.

Doctors may measure triglyceride levels when blood cholesterol score is computed. Generally, a good score for triglycerides is less than 150 mg/dL. Physicians also look at the whole health picture when measuring cholesterol. For example, a person with a family history of high cholesterol or heart disease is more at risk from levels approaching borderline. People with poor diet, extra weight, and a sedentary lifestyle also run greater risk of heart disease from a high cholesterol score.

In most cases when your cholesterol score is borderline, your doctor will suggest a modified diet and an exercise plan. Patients are also advised to quit smoking as this can lower LDL and raise HDL. If the cholesterol score is high, you may need to begin medications to lower the score, while also implementing specific diet and exercise plans to address the condition.

Measure Your Blood Pressure

Blood pressure is measured by the amount of pressure the heart produces to send the blood to all parts of the body. There are two pressures associated with the two sounds heard in everyone's heart. The first sound (S1 or "lub," in lub-dub) is caused by the closing of the mitral and tricuspid valve as the ventricles begin to contract and pump blood into the aorta and pulmonary artery. The second sound (S2 or "dub") is caused when the ventricles finish ejecting, begin to relax, and allow the aortic and the pulmonary valves to close. The "Lub" is systolic pressure and is associated with higher pressure or the number in the score your doctor gives you when he takes your blood pressure. The "Dub" is associated with lower pressure or the number that your doctor gives you when he takes your blood pressure. Normal blood pressure is 120/80. Anything over 140/ 90 is considered high (hypertension). Anything below 90/60 is considered low blood pressure (hypotension).

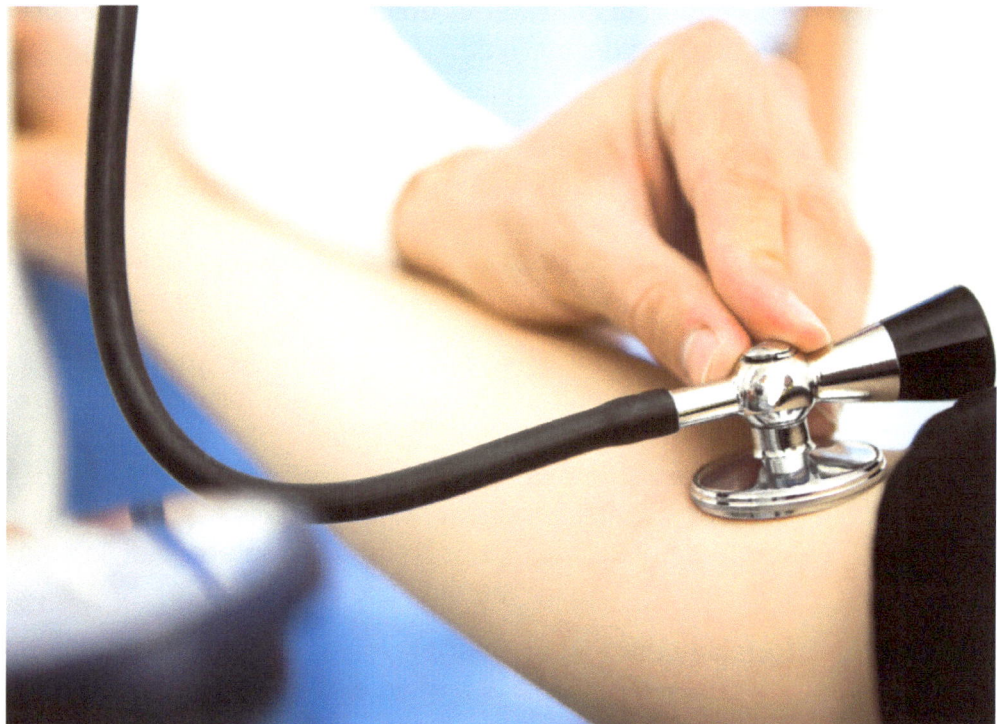

Chapter 6
What To Eat

Over the last 60 years there have been major scientific discoveries that have helped doctors understand the workings of the human body, its organs, and systems. Many of the early healthy eating guidelines on what to eat for improving health were extrapolations of scientific findings of the day. Then, awkwardly, those recommendations had to be rescinded as the true nature of things was discovered. In the 1960s, it was considered unhealthy to eat more than four eggs per week, and today the Harvard School of Public Health (HSPH) suggests that demonization is not all it's cracked up to be. Eating eggs up to 2 times per day is now considered OK. At about that same time, margarine was developed because it was supposed to be better for you than butter, but today we know better. We were told to drink milk for strong bones, eat white bread which builds strong bodies 12 ways, and follow the food pyramid: eat from the 4 different food groups (meat, dairy, fruits & vegetables, and bread). These recommendations proved not to be such a good idea, and we now have a very different food pyramid, which miraculously has turned into a plate. This cycle of scientific breakthrough information, guideline extrapolation, and recommendations turning into misinformation has led most people to be skeptical of what comes out of the scientific studies and has led to ambivalence and confusion about what to do.

During the last 60 years, scientists have had to figure things out blindfolded. Until recently, their ability to see what goes on at the cellular level was not possible. Now, through the development of technology, the blinders have come off, and they can actually see what goes on inside the cells. Technological advances in equipment and procedures have allowed scientists to see down to the 10^{18} power. This scientific revolution gets its rocket fuel from advances in technology, giving scientists the ability to see down to the 10^{21} power. All this is to say that the suggestions that come to us now from the scientific community bear listening to. The recommendation that if you exercise enough and get the proper nutrition you will prevent 70% of all illnesses is based on a clear understanding of what happens at the cellular level in your body.

More than fifteen years ago, the U.S. Department of Agriculture (USDA) created a powerful and enduring icon: the Food Guide Pyramid. This simple illustration conveyed in a flash what the USDA said were the elements of a healthy diet. The Pyramid was taught in schools, appeared in countless media articles and brochures, and was plastered on cereal boxes and food labels.

Tragically, the information embodied in this pyramid didn't point the way to healthy eating. Why not? Its blueprint was based on shaky scientific evidence, and it barely changed over the years to reflect major advances in our understanding of the connection between diet and health.

In 2005, the USDA retired the old Food Guide Pyramid and replaced it with MyPyramid, a new symbol and "interactive food guidance system." The new symbol, basically the old Pyramid turned on its side, has been criticized ever since its debut for being vague and confusing. In 2011, the USDA replaced this much-maligned symbol with a new food icon, MyPlate.

USDA Food Pyramids and guidelines have and always will be bogus. Special commercial interests like dairy, meat, and cereal industries influence how the healthy eating guidelines are written. They obviously want the recommendations to include their products.

As an alternative to the USDA's offering, faculty members at the Harvard School of Public Health built the Healthy Eating Pyramid. It resembles the USDA's pyramid in shape only. The Healthy Eating Pyramid takes into consideration, and puts into perspective, the wealth of research conducted during the last 15 years that has reshaped the definition of healthy eating.

The Healthy Eating Pyramid sits on a foundation of daily exercise and weight control. Why? These two related elements strongly influence your chances of staying healthy. They also affect what you eat and how your food affects you. Whole grains (brown rice and whole wheat pasta too), healthy

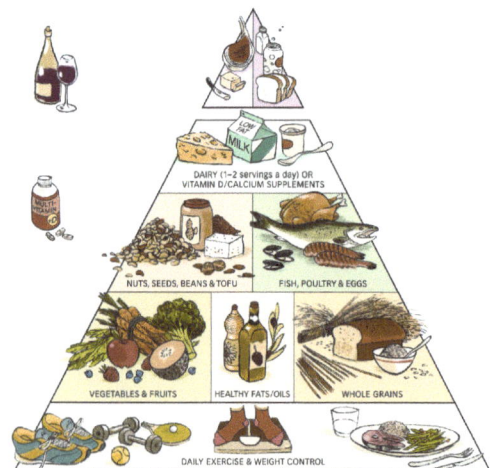

fats and oils (olive, canola, soy, corn, sunflower, peanut, and vegetable oils) and fruits and vegetables make up the next tier of the pyramid. Nuts, seeds, and tofu along with fish poultry and eggs make up the next. 1 to 2 servings of dairy and a vitamin D and a calcium supplement make up the next level of the pyramid. The tip and smallest area on the pyramid suggests that you consume red meat, processed anything, butter, refined grains, white rice, bread, pasta, potatoes, sugary drinks, sweets and salt sparingly.

Scores of studies suggest that having an alcoholic drink a day lowers the risk of heart disease. Moderation is clearly important, since alcohol has risks as well as benefits. For men, a good balance point is one to two drinks a day; in general, however, the risks of drinking, even in moderation, exceed benefits until middle age. For women, it's at most one drink a day; women, obviously, should avoid alcohol during pregnancy.

A new finding from Finnish researchers may lead to specific changes in these guidelines based on a person's blood type. They have proven that blood group antigens on the surface of the blood cells, which determine blood type, serve as an energy source for bacteria in the digestive system. They differ depending on blood type. The blood types have developed from ancient adaptations to food supplies as our ancient ancestors migrated to new geographic regions. The specific antigens serve as a fuel source for specific kinds of microorganisms. People who are overweight tend to have different bacteria than people who are not. In order to optimize the right kind of bacteria in one's digestive system one has to eat the kind of food that promotes the right kind of bacteria for your blood type. Eating the wrong kinds of food for your blood type causes incomplete digestion. This fuels the growth of the wrong kind of bacteria. These unfriendly bacteria produce toxins that researchers have implicated as an underlying cause of weight gain. If you want to get rid of problem bacteria, you have to stop eating food that you cannot digest easily or completely. When people with SIBO (Small Intestine Bacteria Overgrowth) eat for their blood type, the condition fixes itself usually within 6 weeks. (The study was conducted by Finnish Red Cross Blood Service (FRCBS) researchers; results were published in the acclaimed scientific journal PLOSOne Jan 6, 2011.)

Weight loss is not the only benefit of eating for your blood type

The following table outlines the 4 types of blood type and the kind of food people with each type should eat:

Type	Description	What You Should Eat	Avoid
O	High levels of stomach acid help this blood type, which evolved from hunter-gatherers easily process all kind of meat	Lean red meat, lamb, turkey, chicken (not pork), liver, seafood, fish, vegetables, spinach, broccoli, kale, fruit, and iodized salt Grains (on a limited basis)	Beans, legumes, cabbage, brussel sprouts, cauliflower, mustard greens. No wheat products including bread
A	Vegetarian… This type evolved and adapted when human populations began cultivating crops to allow for the optimal digestion of plant foods	Vegetables, tofu, seafood, small amounts of fish, chicken, grains, beans, legumes, fruits, nuts, seeds, cereal and pasta	Red meat, dairy, wheat
B	Type B's are balanced omnivores… descendants of nomadic tribes that raised herds in harsher climates to survive	Lean meat, dairy, yogurt and cheese, vegetables, grains fruit and beans and legumes. Have carbohydrates in moderation	Chicken, corn, buckwheat, wheat, lentil, nuts seeds, and peanuts
AB	Newest blood type… developed when type A's and type B's started to intermingle	Plenty of vegetables and dairy, meat (not red meat) seafood, tofu, beans, legumes, grains, and fruit	Red meat, seeds, corn, buckwheat, and citrus fruits

Weight loss is not the only benefit of eating for your blood type. When one's digestive function is optimized, a wide range of other problems are resolved: problems like internal inflammation, mal-absorption of nutrients, immune system disorganization, hormonal imbalance, fatigue, joint aches, facial rashes, allergies, hot flashes, psoriasis, and other skin problems.

50

Chapter 7
The Science of Supplementation

Maintaining your health, keeping your weight down, and looking your best are easiest when you combine cutting your calorie intake a bit, exercising enough, and having the right blend of nutrients. Proper nutrition revolves around getting enough of the right mixture of nutrients — proteins, carbohydrates, fats, vitamins, minerals, antioxidants, phytonutrients, phytohormones, glycolnutrients — to keep your cells creating energy and working smoothly. Everything needed for proper nutrition is available in the food you eat. There are, however, two problems with that statement:

1. Eating right is not easy or practical for most people

2. If you eat right, you more than likely will take in too many calories

3. The nutritional value from food is no loner adequate

If you want to get the right balance of nutrients, not have to worry about getting too many calories, or eating things that you don't want to eat, you have to take supplements. That is why food supplements are no longer a luxury, but a necessity if you wish to have any hope of a long and healthy life.

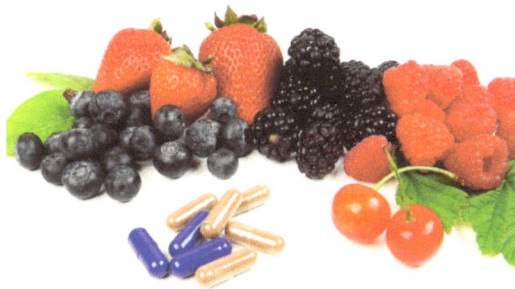

The truth about the food we eat is shocking. The essential nutrients are in limited numbers or are missing altogether. Unfortunately, this is mainly caused by soil depletion as a result of our high-volume overload farming methods. The plants are not getting the nutrients from the soil. To compound the problem, they are also being picked before they ripen (so they have a longer shipping and shelf life). Only fully ripened foods picked from the vine provide the full nutritional value. To further complicate matters, the processing of the food by cooking, canning and drying depletes 90% more of the nutrients. Our bodies are designed to get the nutrition they need for all functions from fresh, raw, natural foods that grow naturally in nutrient rich soil. Those nutrients protect, repair, and regenerate us. If the nutrients are not in the soil, then you are not getting it from the plants that you eat.

Makeup Of Modern Commercial Produce:

- Calories are the same (so you get energy and can gain weight)
- Water content is higher (increases the weight as well as the profits)
- Fiber content is lower
- Phytochemicals (nutrients and hormones from plants like lycopene) are lower to non existent in some cases
- Trace minerals are far lower to non-existent
- Glyconutrients are all gone

Quoting US Senate Document #264 published in 1936:

"The alarming fact that foods (fruits, vegetables, and grains) now being raised on millions of acres of land that no longer contain enough of essential minerals are starving us. No matter how much of them we eat, no man today can eat enough to supply his system with minerals he requires for perfect health... The truth is that our foods vary enormously in value, and some aren't worth eating."

Supplementation of vitamins (especially vitamin C and D), minerals (especially calcium), antioxidants, glyconutrients, essential fatty acids, phytonutrients and phytohormones are mandatory. Only the foolish or the uninformed still believe that we do not need dietary supplements. Science shows that dietary supplementation with the correct nutrients, manufactured with proper quality control and quality assurance, can support the body's physiology effectively. They must also be administered according to guidelines rather than administered randomly. Those that believe that one can get all the necessary nutrients from food alone are

Questions do arise as to the purity and quality of supplements sold

mistaken. For example, you would have to eat more than 100 lbs. of broiled liver or 125 tablespoons of peanut oil for the 500 I.U. of vitamin E that your body requires. (For the 100mg required of lipoic acid, one would have to eat 700 lbs. of spinach.)

Questions do arise, however, as to the purity and quality of supplements sold. 98% of the supplements sold are identical to each other. The only difference is the label. The Quality Control is the same in most cases but Quality Assurance is not. There are thousands of brands of dietary supplements, but only a handful of manufacturers. The retailers rely on the manufacturer to do the Quality Assurance although it should be their responsibility. They do that because it's cost effective. Most companies talk about their quality but the fact is that those statements are based on borrowed data. Even photos, taken at the labs of the manufacturer, are reused and not taken from their own Quality Assurance department.

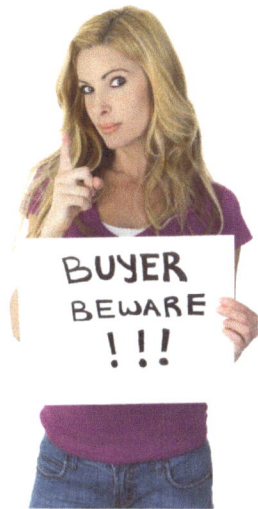

All raw materials must be carefully and repeatedly inspected for pesticides, toxic metals, synthetic chemicals, microbial organisms, as well as the proper blend of vitamins, minerals, phytonutrients (plant nutrients), phytohormones (plant hormones), essential fatty acids (EFAs Omega 6 and Omega 3), antioxidants, and glyconutrients. Farmers throughout the country unknowingly use fertilizer that has at least 17 toxic metals in it. The bottom line: if you need 10 milligrams of something, how you get it isn't as important as getting it active, clean, and pure when you swallow it.

53

Oxygen is necessary for survival but it can be a dangerous friend

Supplements One Needs To Take On A Daily Basis For Optimum Health

There are specific amounts of these that need to be taken and it is not just one specific one, but a combination of all of them.

- Essential vitamins and minerals to create healthy cells
- Antioxidants to protect cells from oxidative damage from free radicals
- Phytonutrients to detoxify the systems (plant nutrients i.e. carotenoids and flavoniods)
- Phytohormones for glandular function (plant hormones, i.e. isoflavones)
- EFA (Essential fatty acids) for cell regulation, hormonal function, and metabolism (improved brain function; reducing depression, schizophrenia, attention deficit disorder, hyperactivity, Alzheimer's disease, and reduction of risk of cancer)
- Essential glyconutrients for cell to cell communication and immune system maintenance and support

Antioxidants

Biological oxidation, the process of making energy (the process that makes all higher life possible), involves moving electrons from one oxygen molecule to the next. The flow of electrons is a vital process that provides the necessary energy for the survival of all organisms. Oxygen, however, can be a dangerous friend. We need ample amounts of oxygen to produce enough energy to survive. We use that energy for growth, physical activity, breathing, thinking, and every other activity that goes on to maintain biological life. Ironically, the production of energy can wreak havoc in the body because it also produces free radicals (free electrons) as a byproduct. Free radicals constantly form almost everywhere in the body and at an astonishing rate. If these free radicals are not quickly trapped, they can cause a great deal of trouble. When electrons are released, they can attack DNA, the genetic material that controls cell

54

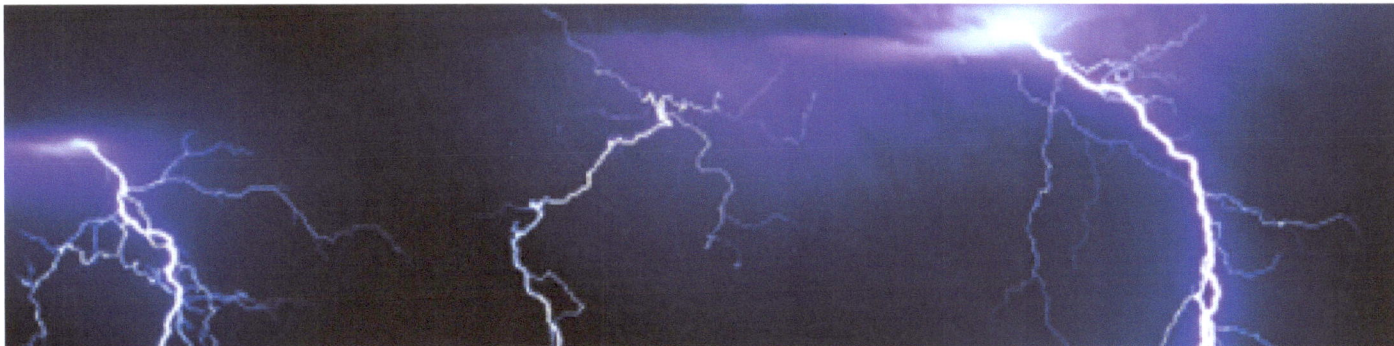

growth and development, which, among other things, can increase the likelihood of cancer. When these free radicals attack fat molecules, low density lipoproteins (LDL) traveling in the blood stream, they set the stage for heart disease and stroke. Scientists now believe that free radicals are causal factors in nearly every known disease, from heart disease to arthritis to cancer to cataracts. Free radicals are also a major culprit in the aging process itself.

> *[Special Note: Most of us, especially when we were kids, have shuffled our stocking feet across a carpet floor in order to give one of your friends or siblings a shock, or maybe you have seen kids with long hair brush it with a dry plastic comb or brush and then it starts to stand straight out. If either of these situations doesn't ring a bell, you surely have seen cloud-to-ground lightning. These situations are examples of free-radical electrons being neutralized. Imagine that in the world of your cells all of your body tissues and organs are constantly attacked by a violent lightning storm.]*

Antioxidants (Free Radical Neutralizers) are needed to eliminate (neutralize) free radical attacks. Antioxidants are a group of compounds produced by your body that also occur naturally in many foods. They quickly trap free radicals before they can escape. Antioxidants work together in your body to maintain your health and vigor well into the later stages of life. They do this by protecting you from damage to your tissues and cells caused by free radical attacks. It was believed that each antioxidant worked separately or independently of the others. It isn't true. There is a dynamic interplay among certain key antioxidants. Dr. Lester Packer, PH.D., has written hundreds of scientific articles on antioxidants and discovered an "Antioxidant Network". These antioxidants are far more powerful together in the correct amounts than they are by themselves. Although there are hundreds of antioxidants, only five appear to be network antioxidants: Vitamin C (500 mg/per day) and 2 kinds of vitamin E (500mg), glutathione (produced in the body), lipoic acid (100mg), and coenzyme Q10 (30mg). What makes them so special is that they work together and enhance the effectiveness of the others. Another obstacle that you will encounter is that you cannot find these in their correct dosages in any of the supplements on the market today.

"Phytonutrient supplements have inert advantages over fruits and vegetables"

Phytonutrients And Phytohormones

Phytonutrients are nutrients concentrated in the skins of many vegetables and fruits, and are responsible for their color, hue, scent, and flavor. Carotenoids and flavonoids, among others, are part of this group of nutrients. To a lesser extent, they are also found in grains and seeds. Examples of foods rich in these nutrients include tomatoes, red onions, green tea, grapes, red cabbage, broccoli, parsley, spinach, raspberry, blackberry, garlic… the list goes on. They are not vitamins or minerals. They are pigments -- or, more precisely, the biologically active constituents of pigments. In the last few years, phytonutrients have been getting greater attention as more and more research uncovers just how powerful these nutrients are for our health. They are potent antioxidants that can neutralize free radicals. Clinical trials are now revealing that phytonutrients can enhance the strength of the immune system and may play a role in preventing certain cancers. Other studies have shown that the phytonutrients in blueberries and blackberries slow brain aging and maintain healthy vision in rats.

Unfortunately, the vast majority of people, especially in the Western world, fall woefully short of following the Healthy Eating guidelines suggested by the Harvard Medical School and, therefore, the right blend of vitamins, minerals, and phytonutrient supplements becomes especially crucial. Indeed, phytonutrient supplements have inherent advantages over certain fruits and vegetables, such as carrots, which can excessively elevate one's blood sugar levels. Because phytonutrient supplements are only the extract of the pigments — where the nutrients are especially concentrated — they are a superior way to derive the best "essence" of fruits and vegetables, without consuming the excess sugars and calories.

Phytohormones are plant derived building blocks that your body uses to create any hormone that your body needs. These substances, also called phytosterols, are vital to a healthy balanced endocrine or hormonal system. Hormones are chemical substances produced by the cells of an organ when you eat food or take supplements that contain these essential nutrients. Your body uses these nutrients to produce the hormones it requires. This is a natural process and there is no synthetic drug or supplement that can mimic this process. The major problem for people

56

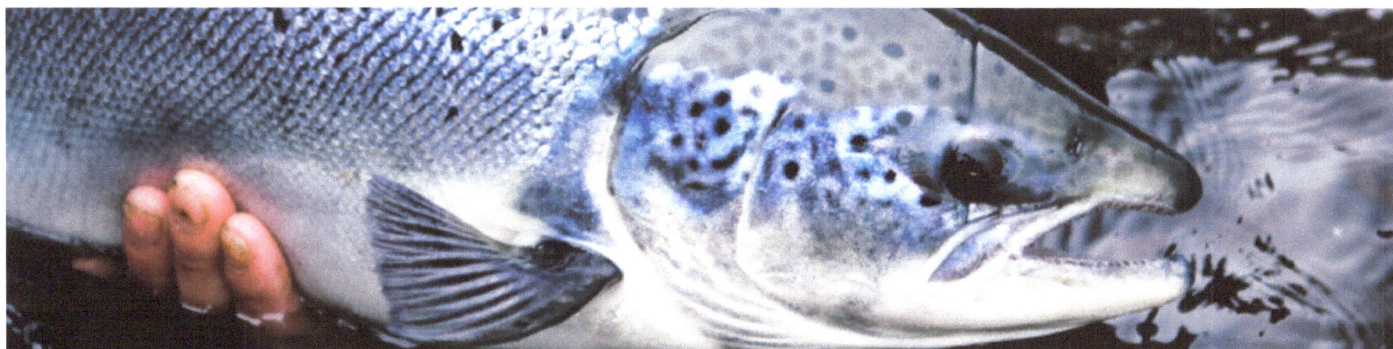

in westernized cultures is that we do not get enough of these essential nutrients from our current food intake, and it is becoming more difficult. Men and women should consume 30-50 mg of these phytosterol plant foods daily. On average we only get 2-4 mg per day, less then 10% of what you must have to balance your body's hormonal system. Hormones can affect many vital functions in your body. That's why keeping your hormones in their proper balance is essential to your health and the way you live. Do you feel tired? Do you have irregular periods? Are you stressed out? How about PMS? Are you low on energy? Do you have early menopause? Or low sex drive? If the answer is yes to any of the above questions, then there is a good chance that your hormonal system is out of balance.

EFA - Essential Fatty Acids

Fatty acids are essential nutrients important for the healthy function of structures and systems in your body. Two very important kinds of fatty acids that are essential for health are omega-6 and omega-3. Unlike other fatty acids that are needed for good health and that are produced in your body, omega-6 and omega-3 fatty acids can only be obtained from your diet. Typically, foods that contain or are prepared with vegetable oils are rich in omega-6 fatty acids, while foods that contain omega-3 fatty acids are rarely available or eaten.

A healthy diet should include a balance of omega-6 and omega-3 fatty acids. Unfortunately, many western diets include too many fried foods, baked goods, cookies, crackers, mayonnaise, salad dressing, and fatty foods that contain unhealthy levels of omega-6 fatty acids. Furthermore, most diets do not include the frequent consumption of fish, leading to an unhealthy ratio grossly in favor of omega-6 (nearly 30:1).

Scientific evidence supporting the health benefits of omega-3 fatty acids is immense. More than 100,000 peer reviewed studies have been published from 1966 – 2004 proving its benefits. Benefits of omega-3 fatty acids include boosting your body's immune system, supporting cardiovascular health, improving joint function and mobility, healthy skin, and normalizing the body's anti-inflammatory response. Omega-3 acts as building blocks for cell membranes of every cell in your body, including brain cells, which help support your brain function.

Nutritional scientists recommend increasing daily consumption of omega -3 to restore a healthy balance of omega-6 fatty acids to omega-3 fatty acids. The best source of omega-3 fatty acid is in fatty fish. There are several problems with that: 1) They don't taste all that great, 2) farmed fish have less omega-3 fatty acid levels, 3) there is a real concern of high levels of toxins and heavy metals present in fish populations. This leaves omega-3 supplements the only practical way of getting your ratios in sync.

Glyconutrients

Scientists have recently discovered a new class of necessary nutrients, certain monosaccharides or carbohydrates that are necessary for maintaining health. These monosaccharides are called glyconutrients and there are 8 glyconutrients essential for each cell in our body to communicate correctly with the next cell or organ. Science has proven that your body uses glyconutrients to prevent infections and disease, and slow the aging process. Since their discovery in 1996, patients with every major category of disease have shown improvement with glyconutrient supplements. Including conditions like diabetes, heart disease, chronic fatigue syndrome, fibromyalgia, hepatitis C, cancer, autism, ADD, ADHD, dyslexia, candida (yeast) infections, asthma, menopause, Tay-Sachs disease, urinary infections, upper respiratory infections, stroke, cerebral palsy, organ transplant, depression, muscular dystrophy, failure to thrive in infants, alcoholism, improvement in antioxidant defense, just to mention a few.

The effectiveness of glyconutrients as the key to proper cellular communication and proper cell function (Cellular Fitness) has been established by the world's leading scientists and researchers. Optimal health is a lifetime commitment. Unlike pharmaceutical drugs that mostly treat symptoms, nutritional supplementation acts as prevention as well

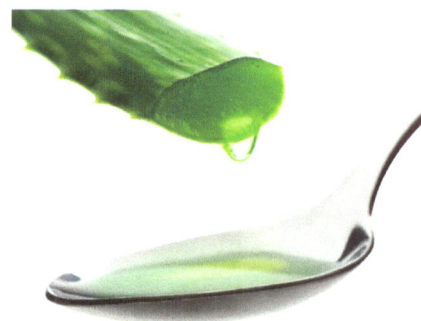

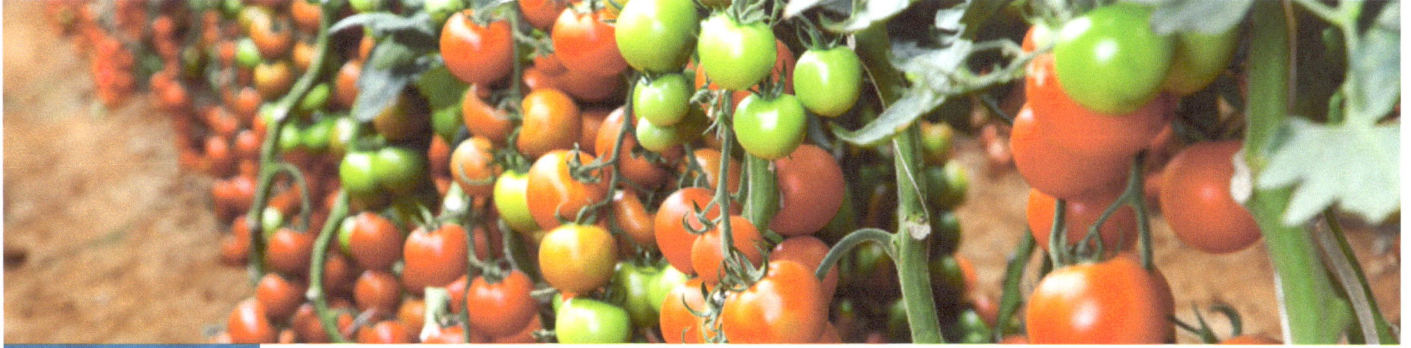

as increasing the body's ability to heal, repair, regenerate, regulate and protect itself.

As we've seen in controlled studies in humans and animals, the saccharides [glyconutrients] in combination with adequate amounts of other key essential nutrients, accelerate healing, improve immune function, slow down aging, improve memory, and lower anxiety without toxic side effects.

So where do you get these rare but necessary ingredients? The best way is from your own "Truck Patch." (This term came from truck's original meaning, "to give for exchange" or "barter. "Truck" then became known as vegetables grown for market). It is homegrown fruits and vegetables that you can pick and eat within 30 minutes.

My dad was the biggest truck patch enthusiast that ever lived. He would plant acres of sweet corn on his hands and knees and plant way too many tomatoes on our farm in Monticello, Minnesota. He would even keep the weeds away by using a hand held hoe. At that time he was in great demand by his students and colleagues. He would schedule appointments between 4 and 7 A.M. for them to sit down with him. Anyone that wanted an appointment after 7 A.M. would have to work in the field hoeing weeds. When I was in high school, my friends and I were hired to paint all the buildings on the farm. One of our additional duties was to tie up the tomatoes so they didn't rot by touching the ground. One day, at break time, we were eating tomatoes and corn until we could eat no more. That is when the tomato fight broke out. It lasted two hours (not including laughing so hard that our sides split and the cleanup). We didn't even put a dent into the number of tomatoes that were still left on the vines. Anyway, the fresh corn that we picked, shucked, and ate and the tomatoes that we picked and ate within ½ hour always tasted so much better than any bought from the grocery store The difference is that the glyconutrients only last about 30 minutes after picking and you can actually taste the difference.

The other way to get glyconutrients is to supplement it from the glyconutrient rich aloe plant.

Chapter 8
What Should I Do?

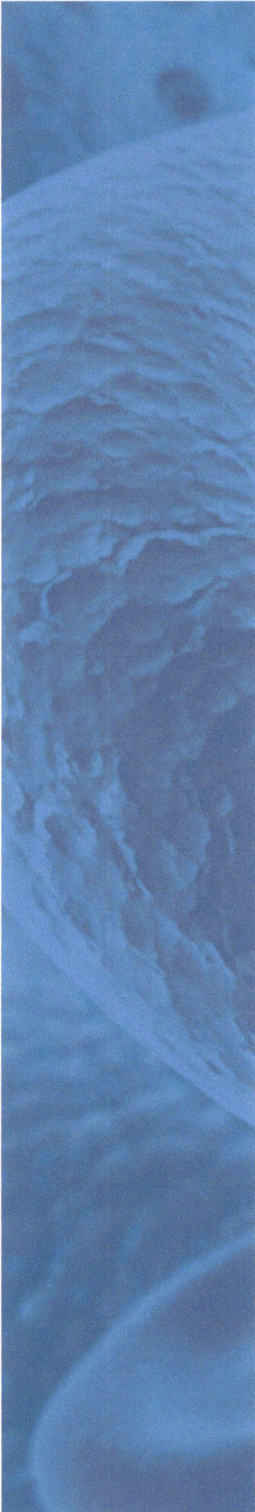

One summer my two daughters (Breezy and Madison), and I were vacationing on the Canary Islands. We were having a wonderful time and decided to go to the beach. All the conditions were perfect except the waves were a little big. My daughter Breezy and I wanted to see if we could body surf the waves. Madison stayed on the beach to play in the black sand. We tried and tried but the waves were breaking very close to shore and it seemed impossible. The tide had started to come in and the waves got a bit bigger, nothing that we couldn't handle. Breezy was 13, a very strong swimmer, and has always been very athletic. As we tried to catch another wave, I noticed that for some reason the waves immediately had doubled from 10 to 20 feet. We were standing at the bottom of the wave and I felt a huge tug at my ankles. I looked up at the wave that was towering above us. I was terrified. We were about to get pounded. I grabbed Breezy by the waist and the wave hit us, held us down for at least 30 to 40 seconds as we tumbled over and over. We both came up just before the next wave hit. I tried to push her to shore as we took our next big breath but the second wave slammed us down again. By this time I only had a hold of Breezy's ankle. Again we came up just before the third wave started to break. After it slammed us, I could not hang on to her any longer. Knowing that I might lose her forever, I dug both my hands and feet into the sand so that the back wash could not take me back into the surf.

That worked. I was out, But Breezy was gone.

I ran back into the backwash and frantically scanned the surface for any sign of her. I was desperate, frustrated, confused, determined, overwhelmed, and I had no time. If I didn't get to her before the next wave, I might never find her!

It surely seemed like an eternity, and there was no sign of her. Just before the fourth wave broke, I saw Breezy pop up out of the surf and she screamed, "Daddy!" At that moment the confusion, frustration, and all the incredible array of emotions had gone and an indescribable calm had come over me. I absolutely knew that I could catch her. She then took a great big breath, and her eyes were as big as dinner plates as the next huge wave hit her for the fourth time. Close to shore I ran and lined up with her. Boom! She was pounded again. The force of the wave sent her right to me. I used the same technique to get out of the water, but this time with one hand and both of my heels dug into the sand. I had a good hold on her with the other. As the water receded, I dragged her up and we dropped to the beach, she was covered with black sand. We both were exhausted and as close to being "drowned rats" as I ever want to be. As she caught her breath she started to cry hysterically. As any parent would know, that was music to my ears.

I don't care who you are or what your circumstances are. You may have been feeling like you are being tossed, tumbled, spun around, and bombarded with an ocean of information to get the results you want. You may be feeling desperate and determined, frustrated, confused, and overwhelmed on how to make fitness and health priorities that fit into your busy life. It may seem like the obstacles are too big to overcome. You can, however, get over under around and through all of these emotions and situations that keep you from the results you want. If you filter through all the options. And stick to what is so. Get rid of the misperceptions, limiting beliefs, marketing BS, temptations, ass-backward exercising methods, hocus-pocus garbage and lies, and stay in touch with the data and facts that come to you from science. You must never give up! Don't let premature aging, decay, and obesity creep into your life. Bring out your best by getting your cells in shape. It will show in your physical appearance (slim, fit, and trim with a healthy glow). If you haven't been exercising, just begin to do something. Stop listening to crap fed to you by advertisers and stop eating their junk. Eat right. Get your nutrition on track. Get the nutrients in the right amounts your cells need to operate properly. Get yourself moving intensively every day. If you have never exercised before, or if you are a world class athlete, the feeling is the same when you exercise intensively. You are just at different levels. If you have been exercising, make sure that the time that you devote to exercise isn't wasted. Make sure that you use the checklist and get all required exercise with the right intensity and duration. Expend enough calories. Measure your output and results. Understand what proper nutrition is and get it.

If you need help getting started on a program go to
www.TheMaxPerformace.com

Again, I don't expect that more than 1 in 1,000 people are going to sit up and get off the couch, but just maybe you're like my friend Ronnie. Ronnie is a painter / kind-of-carpenter. He used to smoke and be overweight, and one day he got a pain in his chest. He didn't think much of it and thought it probably would go away. Then he got it again, and it was more severe the second time. His realization that something bad was creeping into his life motivated him to change his habits. To his credit, he stopped smoking (cold turkey) and joined the gym. He got up and started moving and the pains went away. Once these unnecessary diseases are in your life, it is so much harder to reverse them. It is a lot easier to prevent them.

[Special Note: Even if you do exercise and don't lose weight, there is good news. Although losing weight is one of the main goals, the critical variable is the lifestyle changes. Healthy eating and daily exercise seem to be very beneficial whether they produce weight loss or not. The CDC data support this. Edward W. Gregg, Ph.D., led a team that analyzed data from 6,400 overweight adults. They found that people who tried to lose weight — and do — live longer than those that don't try to lose weight. Unexpectedly and happily, those overweight adults who tried to lose weight — but didn't — had a mortality benefit as well.]

If you have been exercising make sure that the time that you devote to exercise isn't wasted. If you're anything like me, I like to know that the effort I put into something is not classified as "slamming crap against the wall and hoping it will stick." You not only have to put your effort into working out hard consistently everyday but you have to commit to learn the facts, stay up on new developments, and implement what you learn. Look, this is not for everybody. You may be saying to yourself, "But I work out hard every week." I know that you work hard. That is not enough. We all have herd the adage "practice makes perfect." It's nonsense! It's like throwing more crap against the wall. Only "perfect practice makes perfect!" Make sure that you use the checklist and get all required exercise with the right intensity and duration. Expend enough calories. Measure your output and results. Understand what proper nutrition is and get it.

If you need help getting started on a program go to
www.TheMaxPerformace.com

62

Cellular Fitness Checklist
For Optimal Health-Fitness-Nutrition

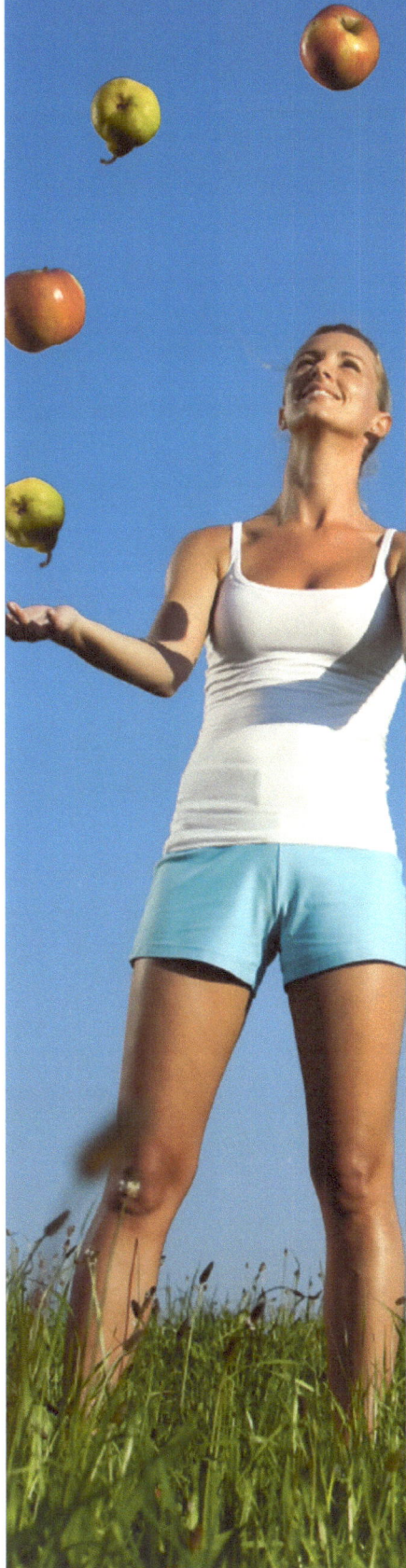

☐ **Exercise Must Be Intense Enough:**

- To expend 2,000 calories per week during exercise at 75% to 85% of maximum heart rate. (Prevention of heart and kidney disease, stroke, high blood pressure, and osteoporosis)

- To change "bad" Cytokines to "good" Cytokines. (Signals growth and stops signals for decay)

- To stimulate the proliferation of Immune System Natural Killer Cells (NK). (Cancer prevention)

- To deplete glycogen stores to stimulate insulin sensitivity. (Prevention of diabetes)

- To lower "bad" Cholesterol (LDL) and Triglycerides and Increase "good" Cholesterol (HDL)

- To lower high blood pressure

- To lower % of body fat

☐ **Exercise Must Be Effective And Efficient In A Short Period Of Time:**

- To increase strength

- To increase strength endurance

- To increase cardiovascular conditioning

- To increase core conditioning

- To increase total body flexibility

- To increase balance and proprioception

- To include plyometrics

- To have a positive improvement in girth measurements and Body Mass Index

- Provide a comprehensive way to get continuous results

☐ **Reduce Injuries While:**

- Exercising
- Preventing falls
- Preventing accidents

☐ **Measure Your:**

- Body Mass Index (BMI)
- Heart rate while exercising
- Calorie expenditure
- Blood cholesterol levels
- Blood pressure

☐ **Use Dietary Guidelines On What To Eat, When To Eat, And How To Get Optimum Nutrition Without Excess Calories**

☐ **Supplement Vitamins, Minerals, Antioxidants, Phytonutrients, Phytohormones, Essential Fatty Acids (EFA), and Gylconutrients**

www.Cellular-Fitness.com

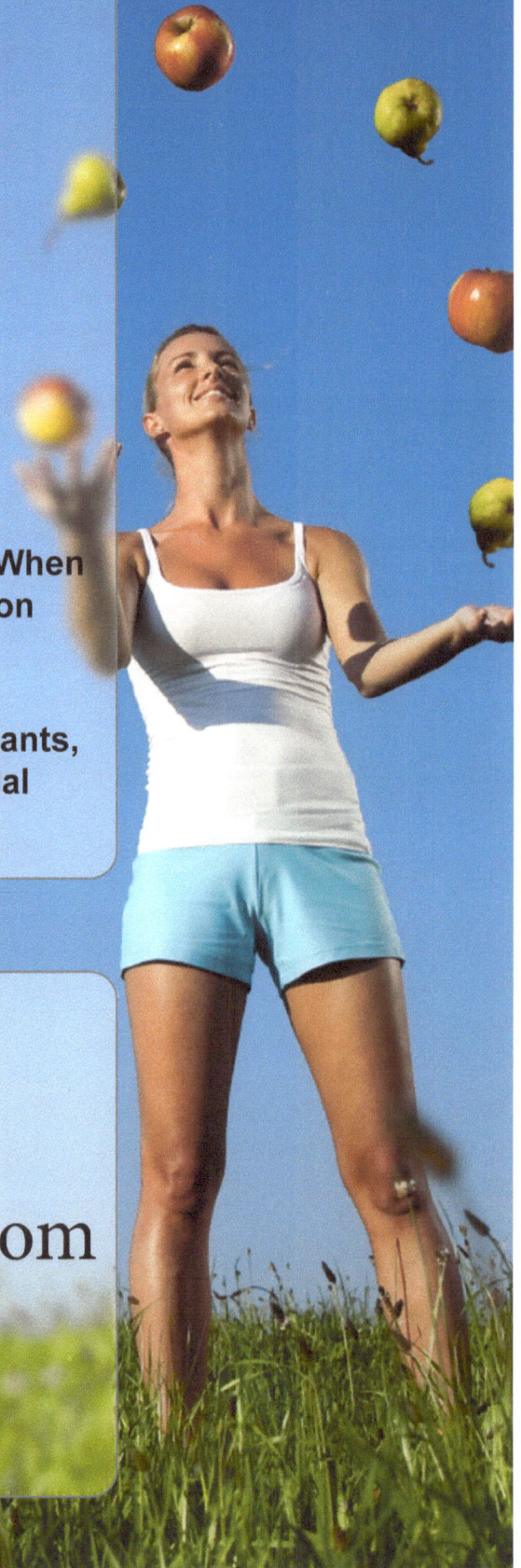

Health-Fitness-Nutrition Blueprint

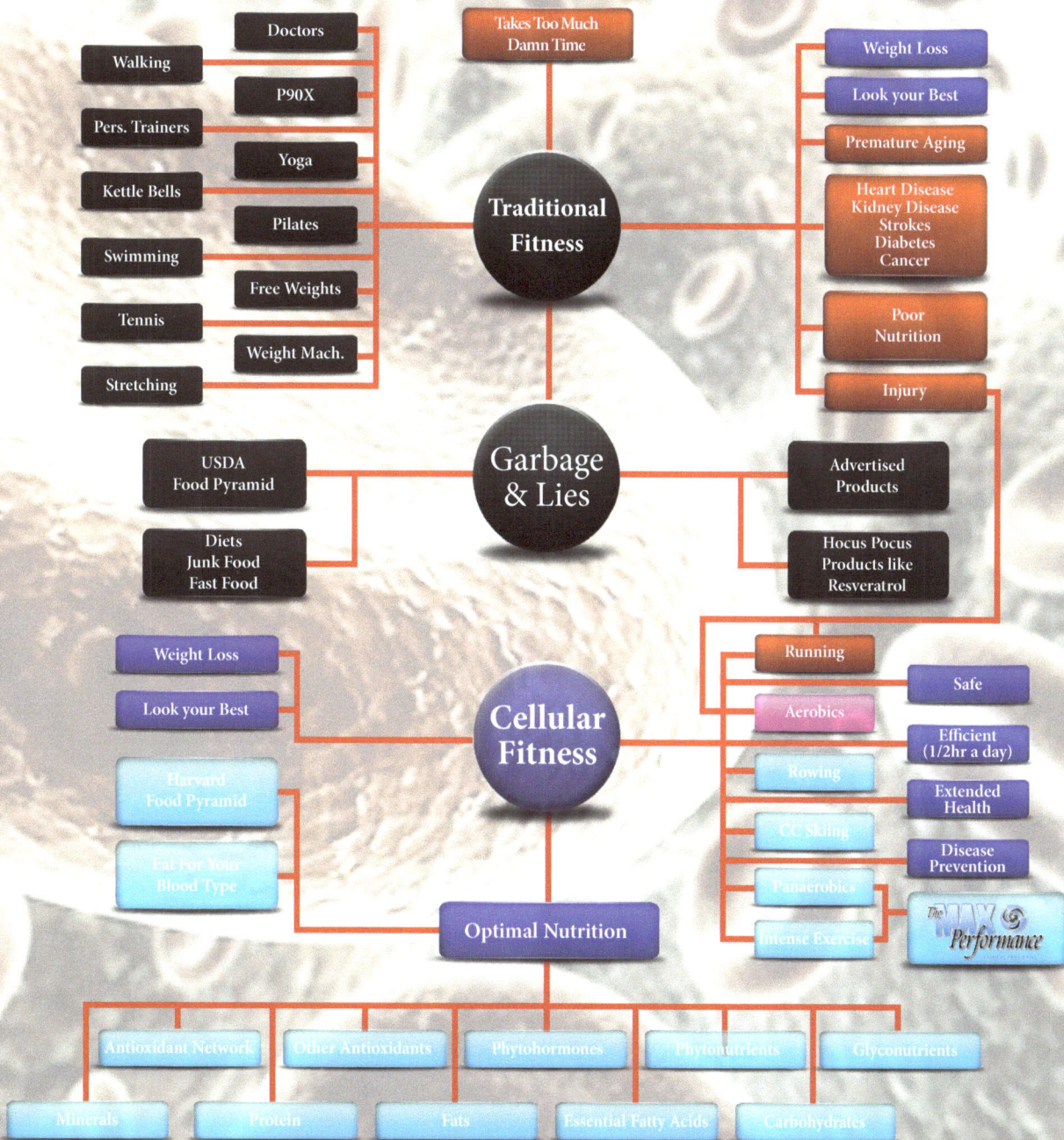

Traditional Fitness

- Walking
- Doctors
- Pers. Trainers
- P90X
- Kettle Bells
- Yoga
- Swimming
- Pilates
- Tennis
- Free Weights
- Stretching
- Weight Mach.

- Takes Too Much Damn Time

- Weight Loss
- Look your Best
- Premature Aging
- Heart Disease Kidney Disease Strokes Diabetes Cancer
- Poor Nutrition
- Injury

Garbage & Lies

- USDA Food Pyramid
- Diets Junk Food Fast Food
- Advertised Products
- Hocus Pocus Products like Resveratrol

Cellular Fitness

- Weight Loss
- Look your Best
- Harvard Food Pyramid
- Eat For Your Blood Type

- Running
- Safe
- Aerobics
- Efficient (1/2hr a day)
- Rowing
- Extended Health
- CC Skiing
- Disease Prevention
- Panaerobics
- Intense Exercise
- The MAX Performance

- Optimal Nutrition

- Antioxidant Network
- Other Antioxidants
- Phytohormones
- Phytonutrients
- Glyconutrients
- Minerals
- Protein
- Fats
- Essential Fatty Acids
- Carbohydrates

Cellular-Fitness.com